THE SECRET LIVES
OF HOARDERS

THE
SECRET
LIVES
OF
HOARDERS

TRUE STORIES OF TACKLING EXTREME CLUTTER

Matt Paxton
with Phaedra Hise

A PERIGEE BOOK

A PERIGEE BOOK
Published by the Penguin Group
Penguin Group (USA) Inc.
375 Hudson Street, New York, New York 10014, USA
Penguin Group (Canada), 90 Eglinton Avenue East, Suite 700, Toronto, Ontario M4P 2Y3,
Canada (a division of Pearson Penguin Canada Inc.) • Penguin Books Ltd., 80 Strand,
London WC2R 0RL, England • Penguin Group Ireland, 25 St. Stephen's Green, Dublin 2,
Ireland (a division of Penguin Books Ltd.) • Penguin Group (Australia), 250 Camberwell
Road, Camberwell, Victoria 3124, Australia (a division of Pearson Australia Group Pty.
Ltd.) • Penguin Books India Pvt. Ltd., 11 Community Centre, Panchsheel Park, New
Delhi—110 017, India • Penguin Group (NZ), 67 Apollo Drive, Rosedale, Auckland 0632,
New Zealand (a division of Pearson New Zealand Ltd.) • Penguin Books (South Africa)
(Pty.) Ltd., 24 Sturdee Avenue, Rosebank, Johannesburg 2196, South Africa
Penguin Books Ltd., Registered Offices: 80 Strand, London WC2R 0RL, England

While the author has made every effort to provide accurate telephone numbers and Internet addresses at the time of publication, neither the publisher nor the author assumes any responsibility for errors or for changes that occur after publication. Further, the publisher does not have any control over and does not assume any responsibility for author or third-party websites or their content.

First edition: May 2011

Library of Congress Cataloging-in-Publication Data

Paxton, Matt.
   The secret lives of hoarders : true stories of tackling extreme clutter / Matt Paxton with
Phaedra Hise.
      p.   cm.
   Includes bibliographical references and index.
   ISBN 978-0-399-53665-6
   1. Compulsive hoarding—United States—Case studies. 2. Obsessive-compulsive disorder. I. Hise, Phaedra. II. Title.
   RC569.5.H63 .P398
   616.85'227—dc22   2011002678

PRINTED IN THE UNITED STATES OF AMERICA

10 9 8 7 6 5 4 3 2 1

Most Perigee books are available at special quantity discounts for bulk purchases for
sales promotions, premiums, fund-raising, or educational use. Special books, or book
excerpts, can also be created to fit specific needs. For details, write: Special Markets,
Penguin Group (USA) Inc., 375 Hudson Street, New York, New York 10014.

I dedicate this book to my wife, Sarah. Very simply, you are everything to me. Thank you for falling in love with a penniless trash man who said he was writing a book. You are an amazing mother and wife and you are gorgeous. I love you.
Matt

For Lily, my junior hoarder.
Phaedra

CONTENTS

FOREWORD

Compulsive hoarding is more than just a hot topic in the media today. It is a long-neglected disorder that plagues millions of people. It is manifested in multiple forms, from hoarding dolls to animals to food, and has multiple causes and outcomes. Hoarding is complex and frustrating for everyone it affects, and it takes away human potential for a safer and more rewarding life.

Hoarding is not a private concern. It affects husbands, wives, companions, parents, children, best friends, neighbors, and animals. It sometimes involves expensive public services, such as code enforcement, fire and emergency services, disability benefits, and legal resources: all supported directly or indirectly by public funds. We are all touched in some way by this growing problem.

Hoarding tendencies often get worse after a traumatic event, and without intercession mild hoarding becomes more severe; it is just a matter of time. Unless someone reaches out to the hoarder, the disorder continues to grow like bacteria in a weakened body. Treating compulsive hoarding is a unique challenge. Unlike other addictions such as using drugs or alcohol, acquiring and keeping objects are behaviors necessary to maintain daily life. It can be difficult to determine when that normal behavior crosses the line into hoarding.

Families of hoarders are often asked, "Why didn't you do something to stop this?" or, "How could you allow your loved one to live this way?" Usually the truth is that they tried and were shut out, sometimes permanently exiled from the hoarder's house. Hoarders often feel threatened, unloved, harassed, and misunderstood; family members feel rejected, ignored, or scolded; neighbors feel annoyed, unsafe, and alarmed. Nobody seems to know what to do.

The Secret Lives of Hoarders is a compelling and compassionate guide to this disorder. Matt Paxton brings understanding and empathy to hoarders and their families who are fighting the battle against clutter, and he knows what it takes to minimize its assault on human life. He is a person of heart and practicality who knows how to reach hoarders and their families. He has learned how to involve public, community, and professional services. He recognizes that hoarders are often victims of an internal process that leaves them helpless when they don't have the benefit of involvement from professionals and a loving, supportive family. He understands the characteristics that hoarders have in common as well as the features that make each case unique. He also knows that, in rare cases, hoarders should be left to live out their lives without intervention—of course, only when health and safety are not an issue.

Matt goes where most people do not dare: inside hoarders' homes. He doesn't shy away from houses defined by squalor and dangerous conditions; rooms filled with rodent-infested debris and no escape from fire; health hazards and falling mounds of clutter; homes that speak volumes of human suffering. There is no direct and simple path to recovery, yet Matt is able to define a process based on his intimate and direct knowledge of a disorder that he has embraced professionally for many years.

In this book you will learn more about hoarding than you would from a professional journal article or scholarly thesis. You will see every aspect of this disorder and its remedies addressed not only from inside the hoarder's world, but also from the point of view of those that hoarding affects.

Matt directly deals with issues about every aspect of hoarding, focusing on real stories that qualify the negative stereotypes and prejudices about people who hoard, and he helps us see that the tentacles of hoarding reach far beyond the person who hoards. It is a societal problem, more so than many other psychological conditions. He takes the sensationalism out of hoarding so that it can be discussed as meaningfully as depression or anxiety. The more we can talk about hoarding in an informed way, the more we can unite resources to remediate it.

Matt writes with concern about the life inside a hoarder's home. He describes the entire spectrum of issues, from what happens in a hoarder's mind to what society can do to help. Inside every hoarder is a person waiting to be released, and this book can be the first step in handling a potentially dangerous disorder from which people lose their lives and society loses valuable human resources. After reading this book, people can look directly at the sad reality of a hoarder who previously mystified, angered, and frightened them. In *The Secret Lives of Hoarders*, Matt is inviting us to embrace hope, join hands, and get the work done.

Suzanne Chabaud, PhD
Clinical Psychologist
Founder of the Obsessive-Compulsive Disorder
Institute of Greater New Orleans

INTRODUCTION

It was the summer of 2006 and I was desperate for work. I was living in Richmond, Virginia, and sleeping on a buddy's couch after a few adventures with jobs that went bad and an attempt to start my own business that failed. I consider myself to be a hard worker and usually have great ideas, but this time I just didn't know what to do.

I decided to try to pick up a few cleaning jobs to earn enough money to help my buddy pay rent. I printed up some flyers and stuck them in mailboxes in an upscale neighborhood, and the next day I got a phone call. An older couple wanted me to empty out their son's house and organize an estate sale. The son, Timothy, had died recently, and they said there was just too much stuff for them to handle.

I agreed to a price of a few hundred dollars. If I had had any inkling what I was heading into, I would have charged thousands. I had cleaned houses before, mostly helping my grandmother and aunts, and I wasn't afraid of mess. But this guy had been collecting things for decades. When his parents showed me into the house, I was overwhelmed by the sheer volume of clutter. Every room had stacks of dust-covered boxes, bags, and cartons piled up to six feet high. Narrow, dark corridors snaked between the walls of stuff—I had to turn sideways to get through some of the tight spots.

On my second day of trying to pull items out of the house to sort and price for the sale, I realized I was in over my head. I called my buddy's brother, Colin, and asked him to help. We needed a truck, so he grabbed another friend who had one. Both of them were still in high school so we were only working late afternoons and weekends. It took us three weeks to finally empty out that house.

Although Timothy had the most cluttered house I had ever seen, the stuff that he'd collected showed that he had a lot of interests, ranging from music to German toy trains to antique furniture. Evidently he went through periods of collecting each one of those, which we could tell by the layers of stuff and the dates on the letters and magazines in the layers. It was like being on an archaeological dig. We could tell that from 1975 to 1980 he was into high-end stereo equipment and vinyl recordings. Then, from 1980 to 1984, he slowed down and was mainly hanging on to mail and magazines. He started saving musical instruments around 1985, and then a few years later added the trains. He collected board games too.

Timothy wasn't there to tell us anything about himself, but we were able to learn a little bit of his story. His parents shared with us that Timothy had killed himself, which made me wonder whether he was one unhappy guy who'd collected all this stuff in an attempt to find some joy in life, or whether his collection had finally overwhelmed him and driven him to despair. Timothy was a mystery that I wanted to unravel.

On the day of the estate sale, I noticed an attractive woman and a companion walking through the house. She kept pointing things out to her friend and explaining what they were. I realized that she knew her way around the rooms, and she recognized everything there. I pulled her aside and asked if she was familiar with the house. She said that she was, and in fact had lived there off and on with Timothy.

It turned out that she and Timothy had been in love for years, but Timothy had never introduced her to his parents because he feared their judgment about being in an interracial relationship. Instead, he guarded a secret life that hid not only his relationship but his ever-expanding collection of stuff. While I didn't press Timothy's friends or parents for much information, the story I pieced together was moving. I saw a grown man, desperately unhappy because he was keeping his life a secret, who had turned to collecting to comfort himself. Then things got out of hand.

That struck a chord with me because I knew a little bit about unhappiness, tragedy, and addiction. I had spent a few months working for a large casino in Lake Tahoe in 1999, and while I was there I fell in love with gambling. It became a full-blown addiction, so bad that at one point I found myself $40,000 in debt. When I couldn't pay my bookie, he broke my nose and I had to leave town.

I eventually paid back my debt and I haven't gambled since, but I know what it feels like to be lonely and miserable, and to turn to something that feels good at the moment but is ultimately destructive. Timothy's situation felt more than a little familiar to me and I found myself wishing I could have met the guy and talked with him about it.

With the estate sale completed and after a final cleanup of what was left behind, I started looking for another messy house to clean.

The second job was referred to me by a social worker in a nearby county. She had a case in which a woman in her mid-forties, Aimee, was living in a terrible state of squalor. She was all but confined to her bed, where she slept, ate, and went to the bathroom by leaning off the side of the mattress. The place had been officially condemned by the county, and since there was some funding to clean it up, the social worker, who had seen a copy of my flyer that said no case was too extreme, called us in. She did give us fair warning that it would really test the limits of our claim. And she was right: The whole place stank from rotting food, urine, and feces. During our first visit to Aimee's house, the social worker gave us the background on this case—and it was the first time I heard the word "hoarder."

I went home and started researching hoarding. The disorder was fascinating because I could relate to a lot of the feelings and experiences that a hoarder goes through. I knew I could really help these people in need.

As my two buddies and I cleaned her house, we talked with Aimee, asking about her life. She admitted that she had rejected everyone because of her hoarding. Although she didn't want us in her home, she was happy to know that someone was interested in her story, and I wanted to find out more about her—and about the phenomenon of hoarding.

Since Aimee, I've had hundreds of hoarding clients, ranging from people who just have a cluttered garage that they want to get under control, to those with entire houses overflowing with trash, feces, animals (alive and dead), and vermin.

I didn't set out to be an extreme cleaning specialist. What hooked me was learning that hoarders are people with serious issues, and that only a few of their life decisions or events separate me from them. What if I hadn't been able to pay back my bookie? What if he had broken more than my nose? What if my friend hadn't loaned me his couch for a few months when I was down on my luck? I could have ended up like any of the clients I work with, or worse.

I have learned that hoarders don't love the way they live. I see them struggling to clean up but just not having the means or the willpower to get it done. Maybe their families don't understand them, or perhaps they have an untreated mental illness that blocks the path to staying clean.

After years of working with hoarders, I've figured out how to make sense of their world because I understand the hard times they've experienced. I can get them talking about their issues and help them straighten out their houses—and their lives. I'm not a therapist, but I work closely with experienced psychologists like Dr. Suzanne Chabaud, who specializes in obsessive-compulsive disorder (OCD) and hoarding at her clinic in New Orleans; Dr. Robin Zasio, who runs the Compulsive Hoarding Center in Sacramento, California; Dr. Lisa Hale, who heads the Kansas City Center for Anxiety Treatment; Dr. Renae Reinardy, head of the Lakeside Center for Behavioral Change in Fargo, North Dakota; and Dr. Elizabeth Moore and other specialists at the Institute of Living in Hartford, Connecticut.

The bottom line is that hoarders are good people who are struggling with difficult issues. To move toward recovery they need love and help, not ridicule. That doesn't mean we don't talk about their issues. Hoarders aren't stupid, and they know that what they are doing is a problem. But threatening, bullying, and issuing ultimatums aren't going to prod them to clean up. They want to de-clutter, but they can't unless they have encouragement and support.

I've worked with hoarders living in houses filled with rotting food and dog feces, and hoarders living with dozens of animals running all over the house. I've helped hoarders let go of their beloved collections of handbags, handguns, and dead rats. The truth is that some recover, and some don't. Hoarding is a serious mental illness, and sometimes "recovery" is a relative term. But I have learned what the challenges are and how to address them. I have seen what the critical elements of success are for any hoarder, and how those elements can combine to give a hoarder the best chance at de-cluttering.

I can help families and others working with hoarders maximize the hoarder's chances for getting and staying clean. It's a long and arduous process, and I will explain how to stay patient and positive for the months, and sometimes years, that it takes.

The key is hope. As long as everyone involved believes that the hoarder's life can get better, it truly can.

Because some of the stories I tell in this book are deeply personal, I have changed the names and identifying details. Some are composites, but all of the stories are true.

WHAT IS
HOARDING?

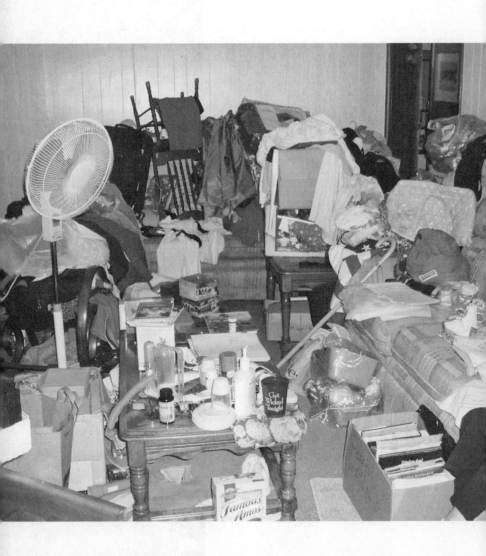

Margaret is a classic, stereotypical hoarder who had clearly given up years ago. Living in a three-bedroom, double-wide trailer home in rural Idaho with too many dogs to count, she had been without electricity or running water for years. The floors were damp with brown muck. Decomposing trash was piled up to five feet high, through which narrow walkways gave limited access to each room.

In the kitchen, flies swarmed the windows and clung dying to a strip of flypaper hanging over the sink. None of the appliances worked except for one microwave that had been stacked on top of a broken one. All of the appliances and cabinets were smeared with unidentifiable black and orange gunk. Dust and cobwebs covered the walls and hung from the ceiling. The bathrooms were just as bad. A bucket of murky water sat next to the toilet, to pour into it for flushing.

The dogs had clawed and chewed away the bottom half of each bedroom door, and they ran through the house and romped wildly on the beds, rubbing their dirty fur around on the bare mattresses. The few chairs were scratched and chewed.

The smell was overwhelming—a mix of urine, rotting food, and dog feces. It was hard to have a conversation over the constant barking. Brown smears coated the walls and windows, and the sagging ceiling had completely fallen in places.

Margaret was a large woman of an indeterminate age, with messy hair pulled back in a ponytail. Every day that we were with her, she wore the same permanently stained T-shirt and shorts, which didn't cover the open sores on her arms and legs. She never smiled or even made eye contact with any of us. She didn't seem to care that she lived in conditions worse than in many third-world countries. Margaret is what most people think of when they think "hoarder."

But there was a time when Margaret wasn't much different from two of my other clients, Brad and Ellen, a middle-class couple raising three small boys in a pretty suburban neighborhood. Ellen was a typical frazzled mom, who got her daily exercise chasing after the kids. Brad was a mellow guy, with dark hair and a little bit of a paunch under his button-down and khakis. The whole family was clean, well dressed, and friendly.

Their house was cluttered—but not the stereotypical place that one associates with classic hoarders like Margaret. There were piles of clothes, toys, papers, and mail that looked like someone meant to get to them a few weeks ago but had gotten distracted.

The telltale sign of hoarders-in-training: The piles were in every room.

Brad worked with computers, and he had saved a lot of his cast-off electronic equipment in the basement, thinking someone might use it one day. Ellen had been a teacher and had kept many of her old supplies and now-outdated workbooks.

Ellen was having trouble keeping up with laundry, with stacks of dirty and clean clothes on the chairs and in front of the washer. The kitchen cabinets were bulging with boxes and cans of food that the two of them liked to stock up on when they were on sale.

Brad and Ellen just couldn't let things go, and weren't processing the avalanche of stuff that comes with raising three active boys. Left unattended for much longer, the clutter would become full-blown hoarding and overwhelm them and their small house.

According to a study by Johns Hopkins University, there are an estimated 12 million hoarders in the United States. Four percent of the population is somewhere in the range of Brad and Ellen to Margaret.

Hoarding isn't about how much stuff a person has. It's about how we process things. Most people can easily make decisions about what to keep and what to toss or donate, and then they follow through. A hoarder can't. There's something off-kilter in the hoarder's brain that we don't fully understand yet. It starts small, and then it gets out of hand.

Hoarding begins like this: Most people who go to a fast-food restaurant and get a cold soda then throw away that big plastic cup when they're done drinking. Maybe they even recycle it. But a hoarder has issues with that cup. The cup is useful. It's a pretty sturdy cup, not a flimsy little paper thing. Maybe a church feeding program or a homeless shelter could use it. Carelessly tossing that cup in the trash would be a waste when there are so many people in this world who can use a good cup. So the hoarder keeps it, intending to get it to the church or shelter. It just never gets there.

Or that cup—decorated with colorful cartoon characters—is meaningful because the hoarder went to the fast-food place with her toddler daughter as a special treat. The moment was an important emotional memory for the mother, and looking at the cup brings back that joyful experience. Throwing away the critical link to such an important occasion is unthinkable.

Hard-core hoarders go through this internal debate with every single item that crosses their path: plastic bags, junk mail, wine corks, fast-food chopsticks, and soy sauce packets.

They are the ultimate recyclers, but for some reason that cycle never gets completed. At some point hoarders lose the stuff-management battle and get overwhelmed. The piles grow, the trash overflows, embarrassment builds, and they stop letting people into their homes. Without help, they have no idea where to even begin to clean up.

Once the possessions start to take over, hoarders tend to get attached to the items no matter what they are. Being surrounded by piles of stuff can be strangely comforting. The stuff is there, day in and day out. It doesn't change, it doesn't leave, it doesn't even move unless the hoarder wants it to. Hoarders feel like they have everything they need—lots of clothing, spare toothbrushes, extra food. They're in the land of plenty where they are in charge and control everything.

SEPARATING HOARDING FROM MESSINESS

Hoarding isn't a character flaw. It's not laziness or forgetfulness. It's a mental disorder. While scientists and medical professionals are still figuring out exactly what hoarding is and what causes it, most agree that it is a glitch in the brain that manifests itself by making a person want to hang on to things, whatever those particular things may be.

The critical thing is how to determine if someone is just messy or a bona fide hoarder. Everyone builds up a few piles now and again, and many of us have a growing "collection" of something like porcelain Christmas houses or old *Sports Illustrated* magazines. When is that a problem?

Hoarding is an issue when the clutter begins to affect the activities of everyday life: cooking, cleaning, entertaining, and moving freely about the house. In the early stages it can be difficult to tell hoarding from messiness. Someone who shuffles piles of junk mail around the kitchen counters or who is too embarrassed by a messy house to invite people over might just be on the slippery slope to hoarding—or not. If the clutter gets progressively worse instead of better, it's probably hoarding.

THE HOARDING SCALE

Appreciating how serious the issue is—or could be—means understanding where the hoarder fits on a scale from mild to totally dysfunctional. Quantifying and qualifying the problem will then help guide what actions need to be taken to aid the hoarder.

Created by the Institute for Challenging Disorganization, which is dedicated to the benefit of people affected by chronic disorganization, the Clutter Hoarding Scale is an organizational assessment tool for use by organizational professionals. It ranks hoarders from Level 1 (Brad and Ellen are the closest example discussed in this book) to Level 5 (like Margaret), depending on what's in the house and how it's being maintained.

To me, hoarding is as much about the individual as it is about the stuff. This scale does not take into the account the physical health of the individual or the person's mental state. So, as shorthand for working with hoarders, I developed my own version of this scale.

The original scale that my company, Clutter Cleaner, used was a pretty subjective one and based roughly on the number of dead cats we found in a house. But after years of working with hoarders we've refined our own language and now incorporate not only what we discover by way of stuff but also the physical and mental status of the client. As well, the Clutter Cleaner scale takes into account the social factors of American society, in which we have a lot more leisure time, and the pressure that everyone—not just hoarders—is under to consume.

The Clutter Cleaner scale is not used by psychiatric professionals or therapists. We use it as a guideline to help understand the hoarders with whom we work and to determine how much we can realistically expect them to change.

▶ Stage 1

Brad and Ellen represent fairly typical Stage 1 hoarders. Their clutter wasn't excessive. Their house had all doors and stairways accessible. All the members of the family were healthy, clean, and well nourished, including the dog. Brad and Ellen both participated in a few hobbies, maintained their finances, and regularly invited friends and family over. Ellen felt a little anxious about the clutter, but it didn't affect their lives in a major way except for having to move piles around the house.

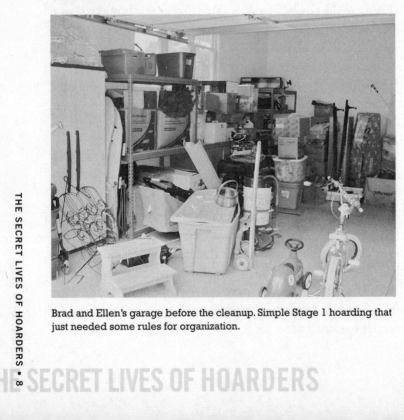

Brad and Ellen's garage before the cleanup. Simple Stage 1 hoarding that just needed some rules for organization.

A Stage 1 hoarder usually isn't recognizable as a hoarder. At this stage, the problem isn't about volume; it's more about the habits that the hoarder is developing as he or she tries to handle clutter. Early-stage hoarders have trouble parting with items and are beginning to build collections. They may be starting a shopping habit or a hobby that lends itself to acquiring things. The clutter will grow and hoarding will develop if these behaviors aren't curbed.

For example, Brad's computer parts could easily accumulate to the point at which they become too much to deal with. Or they could take on more emotional value than physical value, so he'd be reluctant to just toss or recycle them. Ellen risks getting behind in her general cleanup—especially things like laundry. Clothes might become unusable and she'd have to buy more—often of the same things—just to make do. And the more stuff one has to cope with the harder it is to keep the dust, dirt, cobwebs, and whatnot at bay.

Although messy, Brad and Ellen's house had a clean kitchen and bathrooms, and everyone in the family was still able to wash and get clean clothes daily. Brad and Ellen were apologetic about the growing mess, but they were relatively happy, without a lot of anxiety about the situation. More important, they were self-aware enough to get help at an early stage.

▶ **Stage 2**

Coping with stuff is like filing, before the days of the "paperless office." You leave it for a day or two, you can cope. After a week it becomes a pain but manageable. In a month or two, you are ready to give up and stuff the whole lot under your desk. After all, if you didn't need the papers for a month or however long they sat in a pile, how important could they be anyway? And this thinking—or inaction—is exactly what leads to Stage 2.

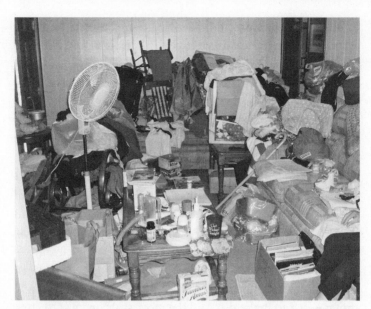

Typical Stage 2 family room. The furniture is starting to disappear under the stuff, but the room is still functional and pathways exist.

If Brad and Ellen hadn't sought some help early on, their house could soon have faced some safety issues, where an exit from the house is blocked, or there's one room that's basically an uninhabitable dumping ground. Everyone has a junk drawer that holds odds and ends of stuff. When that junk drawer becomes a junk room, it's a signal that you are moving up to another stage. Or if a major appliance like a dishwasher or air conditioner hasn't been working for several months because it's difficult to get to it for repair, it is most definitely a sign of a Stage 2 hoarder. And along with this, there is less attention to housekeeping: Dishes pile up in the sink and shelves remain dusty. If there are pets, there may be some odor from a dirty litter box or one too many accidents.

Hoarders at this stage are starting to focus more on clutter than on life. They tend to invite fewer people to their homes from a sense of embarrassment, which is exactly what happened to Jackson.

Jackson hoarded items having to do with the rock group Blondie. He collected every bit of memorabilia he could find with Blondie's name on it, from music to souvenirs. His house was very clean; he had his collection carefully cataloged and arranged. But it was overflowing out of the two rooms he had dedicated to be more or less the "museum." At some point, Jackson had stopped being discriminating in his collecting and it practically drove him out of his house.

Emotionally, there is some anxiety and mild depression at this stage. A Stage 2 hoarder begins to withdraw from friends and family. As a substitute, he or she begins to acquire more things to fill that void, and the cycle continues in earnest. As the hoarder brings home more items, managing those takes priority over personal relationships. At this point, the hoarder begins to shift from embarrassment to justification, explaining why he or she "needs" the possessions.

▶ **Stage 3**

It is at this stage that the signs of hoarding become evident to the outside world. There may be a little structural damage to the house—for example, a sagging porch. Some indoor items are stored or tossed outside. There's some evidence of what I call "spaghetti" extending all around the house— tangles of power cords and phone lines jury-rigged to keep things operating when electrical outlets are blocked off. If there are pets, there are also some carpet stains and fleas. The sink is usually filled with dishes and standing water. Walkways and stairs are overtaken with clutter and difficult to navigate. Outside storage—a garage or shed—overflows.

Stage 3 hoarders are losing track of their personal care— bathing and haircutting aren't a priority. Because kitchens at this stage are often borderline functional, Stage 3 hoarders tend to eat food that's been cooked/reheated in the microwave oven or fast-food takeout. This almost always causes

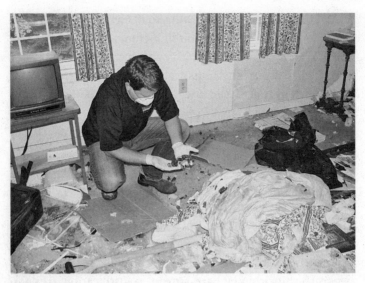

Matt sorting through a Stage 3 animal hoarder's living room, trying to find family jewelry among the dog feces.

weight gain. For Stage 3 hoarders, physical activities are often limited. They'll sit for hours in front of a TV or computer screen. The bad food and lack of exercise contribute to the weight gain, and the classic stereotypical picture of the hoarder emerges. The Stage 3 hoarder's pathology is slipping into the workplace, and job performance suffers. Plus finances are probably becoming an issue.

At this stage the hoarder is often depressed and claims to want to be left alone. Many hoarders find their best companions in their pets—and often enter into another type of hoarding. (More on animal hoarding follows.) It's likely that family members have tried to clean the house and were either rejected or withdrew, their attempts in vain.

▶ Stage 4

At Stage 4, there's structural damage to the house in several areas—floors and ceilings may be sagging, or there is unrepaired water damage. There may also be mold, spiderwebs, and bugs. There's rotten food in the kitchen. Major appliances don't work and can't be accessed for repair. Things are stored in odd places: clothes hang from the bathtub curtain rod; important documents are in the oven. This house is truly dangerous, with blocked exits, poorly stored chemicals, and papers creating a real fire hazard.

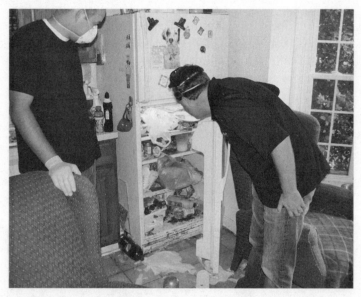

Cracking open a refrigerator like this one, which hasn't been open in more than fifteen years, is one of Matt's and his crew's least favorite jobs.

The Stage 4 hoarder begins to retreat to a small area of livable space in the house—a "cockpit" where the hoarder spends most of his or her time. The hoarder probably doesn't do laundry, and just buys clothes at the thrift shop to replace soiled shirts and pants. A hoarder at this stage may bathe at the sink or not at all.

Hoarders have pretty much stopped following societal rules at this stage. They struggle to get to work on time, or they may quit working and be unable to pay the bills. The phone may be ringing frequently from bill collectors—until it too is shut off, along with the electricity and water. Pets are beginning to be on "vacation," which means either dying or running away. Because their lives look so bleak, Stage 4 hoarders talk mostly about past memories or unrealistic plans for the future.

▶ Stage 5

Margaret is a Stage 5 hoarder, which is as bad as it gets. There is major structural damage to the house, with severe mold, strong odors, bugs, rodents, and cobwebs taking over. Entire floors of the house might be completely blocked off. There are walls of clothes or other items in every room. The hoarder spends the entire day struggling to complete simple tasks like eating, sleeping, and going to the bathroom. Diet is generally limited to soft drinks and either fast food or now-expired generic brand food that was bought on sale.

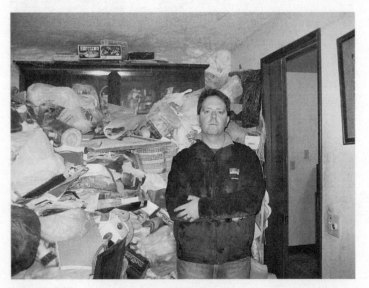

Typical of the "great walls" of clutter that Matt and his crew encounter in the most dangerous Stage 5 hoarding cases.

If friends and family are still in contact with the hoarder, they are deeply concerned and have probably tried interventions. A hoarder at this stage is usually in serious financial trouble, and it's likely that someone has contacted city or county authorities.

Depression is often so severe for a Stage 5 hoarder that he or she struggles to get up each day. A hoarder at this stage is often confused, perhaps saving items for people who are no longer living. Hoarders at this stage don't leave the house, with the exception that some may move to their cars or a homeless shelter to sleep.

None of these stages is clear-cut. The scale shows a continuum in which a Stage 4 hoarder could have a clean house with no bugs or cobwebs, but it is so packed with stuff that nothing is accessible. Or a Stage 2 hoarder might have a fairly accessible house but a completely filled basement and attic.

The initial assessment of what is being hoarded and where the hoarder is on this scale gives us a sense of the severity of the problem. And while it seems, on the surface, a simple matter to call in a cleaning and repair crew, dealing with hoarders is far from simple. The key to a successful cleanup is to understand what makes hoarders do what they do.

WHO ARE THE HOARDERS?

When I first started my business and was searching for jobs, I would drive around and hunt for hoarders. I looked for a house where the blinds were closed and pressed against the windows. Or the yard was overgrown and animals were roaming around. I knew that I'd find a likely client if stuff was piled on the porch or in the yard or in an outbuilding on the property. The stereotypical hoarder—the overweight, elderly woman, unkempt, dressed in layers of clothes, sitting in front of the TV all day long—lives in that house.

Well, at least that's the stereotype. But in the years since I started Clutter Cleaner, I've worked with hundreds of hoarders of every stripe. The truth is that hoarders come in all sizes, shapes, colors, ages, and backgrounds. Many of them contradict the stereotype: They're smart, educated, and have good jobs. If you met them at work or in a social situation, you would never guess they were hoarders. Unfortunately, this makes it easy for outsiders to minimize or dismiss the problem.

Margaret actually seemed to fit the classic type—the older, poor woman living in squalor with her pack of dogs. Hers was a full-blown case in which hoarding had destroyed her house to the point that the living conditions were completely unsafe.

By contrast, Brad and Ellen's house didn't look like a typical hoarder situation, but it had become an issue for them because the clutter was making it difficult to keep track of toys and clothing, and they felt embarrassed by how it looked. More important, how to deal with the clutter had started causing arguments that were spilling over into other parts of their marriage. They called me for help because they sensed that if they didn't address it, the mess (and their bickering) would keep spiraling out of control.

When I first met Li outside her house I would never have guessed that she was an extreme hoarder . . . and neither would anyone else, since she hadn't let anyone except for two of her five children into her home in years. In her mid-sixties, Li was generally well dressed, tastefully made up, and in good shape. She looked in every way to be a pampered suburban housewife, but she was, in fact, a Stage 5 hoarder.

Li and her late husband had raised five children in their four-thousand-square-foot, three-story farmhouse in rural Connecticut. My first visit to Li's home revealed that the house and the barn on the property were all completely stuffed to the gills with clothing and household items. Li was pretty well confined to her kitchen and adjacent bathroom, hemmed in by the massive amount of stuff that she had purchased during more than a decade of hoarder-fueled shopping.

Li's house was big enough so that she had room to save all of her now-grown children's clothes and toys, which is what was at the bottom of the piles. And when her husband died and the children had moved away, Li started filling up the house in earnest.

And then there's Rick, a tenured college professor who could excuse his saving papers, magazines, journals, and other printed matter—until it got of out of hand. At school, Rick appeared to be just a regular guy, neatly dressed, articulate, and rational. When he talked about his hoarding, he could almost convince people that saving every scrap of information he came across was a natural extension of his job. But one look inside his house revealed that instead, his hoarding was making his living conditions unsafe. His house was a firetrap.

Like Rick, Jackson was a well-educated person with a good job. By all accounts he was good at his job as a social worker—he even sometimes worked with extreme hoarders. Jackson was young, healthy, in good physical shape, and kept his small house clean and orderly—at least until his Blondie memorabilia collection gradually took over, like so much kudzu. He was able to convince himself—and others— for a long time that he didn't have a problem even though he'd stopped having friends over to visit because he was embarrassed by the clutter. His collection may have sounded like an interesting hobby to outsiders, but it was ruining Jackson's life. But he couldn't get it together enough to tackle the ever-growing mounds of stuff.

Katrina was a retired divorcée who had worked as an office manager for a large company. She was an energetic redhead, smart and opinionated, whose hoarding started with a home-based business selling skin care products. She was storing an ever-growing amount of samples, catalogs, awards, paperwork—and lots of inventory. In addition, years earlier, Katrina had been so determined to get a decent settlement out of her divorce that she actually went to law school and got her degree. Now, long after the settlement, Katrina still had boxes, stacks, and filing cabinets full of legal paperwork. Katrina argued that these were very important documents, which they may have been, but she didn't really need to hold on to everything so long after her divorce was final. At the very least, this stuff didn't belong in her living space. She could have scanned or stored most, if not all, of the data. As a result, after years of neglect, mold was evident along the walls, floors, and baseboards of her home. She even had ivy growing through the floor in one of her rooms.

Someone like Margaret looks like a hoarder—overweight, straggly hair, socially withdrawn, and living in a messy house. Because of that she is more likely to get attention and help from friends, relatives, or social services. But hoarders like Li, Rick, Jackson, and Katrina can slip under the radar, with their problem growing worse until it threatens their relationships, their livelihoods, and their health.

It's impossible to diagnose hoarding solely based on what someone says, what they look like, or even what shape the house is in. Brad and Ellen were smart, social people and their house wasn't so messy that a visitor would assume they had a problem.

It makes sense how hoarders like Li start collecting stuff. But how do things get so out of control? Katrina was clearly an intelligent person who knew that mold is dangerous. Why couldn't she stay clean? These are frustrating questions that many family members and friends of hoarders ask, and the answers aren't always simple.

WHAT HOARDERS HOARD

When people think of hoarders, they think of someone living among broken furniture, decomposing garbage, and animal feces. But hoarding isn't just about dirt and trash; it's about hanging on to things that seem important for one reason or another. The rest is garbage that accumulates because everything else has gotten out of control.

Most hoarder houses end up looking like the owners collect general clutter—too many old clothes, sheets and towels, tote bags, warehouse-sized crates of food, and other items from daily life. Yet some hoarder houses are pristine and packed with fine antiques and collectibles. Most often the hoarders start with that sort of thing, be it magazines, clothes, or valuable artifacts, which then accumulates and takes over the house. The tendency to hoard *one thing* often spreads until the hoarder becomes incapable of getting rid of *anything*.

I've seen homes and yards full of bicycles, airplanes, pornography, empty prescription bottles, live birds, dead rats (carefully sealed in plastic bags), handbags, and even a collection of ten thousand cookie cutters. Hoarders are as diverse and creative as the stuff they collect.

▶ The Animal Rescuer

Margaret was a Stage 5 dog hoarder. She started out with one dog, but her love for animals quickly made her the go-to person for strays. Margaret's dogs had complete run of the house, chewing, eating, and marking anywhere they liked and sleeping in a pack on the beds. Her animal hoarding eventually extended to a few parakeets in a large cage and then to ten horses she kept in a barn behind the house. Margaret was unable to say no to any animal in need.

The classic stereotype of the animal hoarder is the old lady with too many cats, like our client, Rose, whose thirty or so cats roamed freely through her house and garage. During the time I worked with her, every time I tried to breathe without a face mask I got a mouthful of fluffy hair. My crew and I found more than fifty dead cats and kittens; their dried-out skeletons were flattened under piles of clothes and boxes.

Rose never noticed any missing pets because there were just too many around to keep track of. The decaying animal smell didn't get anyone's attention because the whole garage and house reeked of cat urine.

Ironically, Rose wanted to protect and care for the animals, but her hoarding got in the way. The animals quickly became endangered simply because she couldn't feed all of them regularly, change their litter, and provide adequate living conditions.

It's hard for a non-hoarder to understand why someone needs so many pets. In so many cases, it became clear to me that a hoarder overlooks the mess when the animals are a comforting substitute for human contact. An animal that loves and doesn't judge might be the only positive thing in a hoarder's day. And taking in animals that would be neglected otherwise gives meaning to the hoarder's life. It can be really empowering to feel so important to the very survival of another living being, but even those best intentions go horribly wrong.

▶ The Information Junkie

Rick, the college professor we met earlier, had twenty-five years' worth of mail, magazines, and financial documents. A two-foot-thick layer of compressed paper carpeted the whole house.

Every surface in Rick's house was covered in mail. The living room was so cluttered with huge piles of paper and other items that we didn't realize there was furniture in there

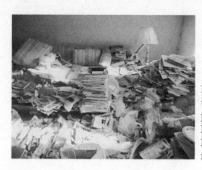

It is difficult for most "information hoarders" to let go of newspapers, books, or mail. Matt has learned that many hoarders know where a specific issue of a magazine or paper can be found.

until we cleaned it up. Rick had spent his whole career gathering, sorting, and sharing information, so for him to throw away that paperwork was almost sacrilegious.

This is a form of information hoarding. Rick couldn't bear to let information slip through his fingers, out of his control. Books, newspapers, CDs, magazines, photographs—basically any printed or recorded material was important to him. Information hoarders are usually people who have dedicated their careers, and lives, to education in one form or another. Many of them are highly educated themselves and work at top-level jobs in government, law, corporate America, or at universities.

The average person will read the morning paper and then toss it into the recycling bin. Rick read it and then decided that the article on investing would be really helpful one day. Or he'd save a magazine with a gardening article for a friend. (Of course, the friend inevitably did not get the magazine.) Then there were the crossword puzzles—so good to take to a doctor's appointment and work on in the waiting room. So each newspaper or magazine went into a pile. But the next day another newspaper went on top of the growing stack, and pretty soon he had years-old piles of paper that he saw as full of potentially useful information and entertainment.

The logic that so much information can be stored online nowadays has little effect on information hoarders. Some hoarders do, in fact, use their computers to back up the

THE SECRET LIVES OF HOARDERS

physical items they are holding. But for many hoarders, "online" can seem nebulous. If it's not in the house, hoarders worry that they can't locate what they need instantly. Surprisingly, information hoarders can usually find what they're looking for—or at least know where it is in the piles, though it may be buried three feet deep.

▶ The Shopaholic

Marcie's house was packed floor to ceiling with unopened plastic bags of items from discount and big-box stores. This stout, gray-haired grandmother who dressed in flowery polyester pantsuits loved to shop. Her hoarding had progressed to the point where she'd go shopping to replace things she couldn't find in her mess, but then she would also buy extra stuff while she was at it. For years, Marcie would come home from her latest spree, put her shopping bags down on the nearest pile, and then never look at them again. Soon she forgot what she had just bought and often ended up buying replacements for something she didn't know she already had—something still pristine in its original packaging.

Marcie just couldn't pass up a good bargain. She got a real "high" from the hunt-and-purchase process and couldn't stand the thought of a good sale item going to waste. She appreciated the value of that sale item and felt smart for grabbing it.

There's a reason why shopping has become what's called "retail therapy." When Marcie bought yet another dress for her three-year-old granddaughter, who already had way too many dresses, Marcie wasn't thinking about the dress. She was thinking about the granddaughter: how cute she was, how she would love the dress and smile lovingly at her grandmother with those big dimples. Marcie might have been thinking about how she would have loved to have had a dress like that when she was three. And she was thinking that maybe her family would love her again if she gave the beautiful dress to the granddaughter.

In this case, the dress is really a stand-in for human interaction. And in fact, the dress probably won't ever get to the child. It will go on top of the pile of other shopping bags filled with gifts. Once Marcie got home, the rush was over, and she didn't follow through.

This high is just like what a junkie feels when doing drugs. Marcie was replacing deep-seated negative memories with short-term positive feelings through consumption. But the quick hit of happiness she got from buying would never fix the sadness from the past. The shopping high was enough to get Marcie through an afternoon, or maybe even a day. But that's the scariest part of hoarding—the deeper someone like Marcie gets into it, the more often that person needs a shopping-happiness boost.

▶ The Do-It-Yourselfer

Lucy was a crafter whose rooms were filled with four-foot-high piles of yarn, fabric, candy-making molds, Wilton cake pans, and baking accessories—and only narrow passageways gave her access through the house. Until she retired a couple of years earlier, she was an accountant, but her real love was making fancy cakes on commission from her friends and coworkers for birthdays and holidays. She was also a master maker of crocheted blankets and handmade holiday ornaments. When we met up with Lucy, her house was clean, just packed with unlimited craft supplies.

With her short hair styled and colored, decked out in matching pants and sweater sets, Lucy had lots of energy and was so engaged in many interests that she belied her seventy-one years. In spite of the clutter in her house, she didn't fit neatly into the Stage 2 hoarder profile. Lucy's daughter had called us for help, and Lucy agreed to have us clean. She was very personable and seemed genuinely happy to have our cleaning crew come to her house. When we arrived, she was thumbing through a pile of craft magazines and talking about the afghans she still intended to make. (I call these the "fixing to's," as in "I'm fixing to make that blanket.")

We sorted through her craft items and discovered that she had at least fifty cake pans and more than nine hundred rolls of yarn. She used about eighteen rolls of yarn to make each blanket, which took her about three months to crochet. At that rate, if she never bought yarn again, it would take her *twelve and a half years* to use up all that yarn. Of course, that doesn't account for the time needed for making cakes and other crafts, or for new hobbies or pastimes.

Do-it-yourselfers are distinguished from other hoarders by the emphasis they put on *future plans*. It sounds reasonable that a crafter would need a good supply of fabric or yarn, or a hobby mechanic would need a load of spare parts. Most DIYers buy ahead—on sale or when supplies like used parts become available. But the crafters and hobbyists who slip into hoarding are generally suffering from the "fixing to" blues.

While DIY work is rewarding, and it's exciting to try lots of different things in life, at a certain point there's just not enough time to do everything. Mechanics can easily turn into hoarders as they collect parts and cars that they plan to restore. One car project is enough to keep anyone busy for a long time, and in the meantime a hoarder's collection of items for future projects grows and grows. These hoarders are usually unable to focus on completing a project because they are distracted by plans for so many others.

Craft hoarders are usually very talented and receive a lot of compliments on what they make. Lucy's cakes were amazing, and she got a lot of positive reinforcement for that, which made it easier to justify collecting her pans and decorating supplies.

At some point, DIY hoarders switch from focusing on the actual compliments to *perceived* compliments. Those are the compliments that they know they will get when they finish a project. They skip right over the step of actually making anything and instead just collect supplies and give themselves lots of positive reinforcement with those imagined compliments.

After retirement, Lucy wasn't making cakes anymore. But she continued buying pans and accessories. The mind game in which she was engaged made it very difficult for her to part with her baking tools, for example, because letting those go meant giving up the anticipated rewards—by way of compliments and recognition—that she hoped to get, no matter how unrealistic her expectations might have been.

▶ The Collector

Jackson, a tall, muscular, and well-dressed man in his late thirties, always made eye contact when he talked, a skill that he used effectively in his job as a city social worker. To the outside world, Jackson seemed confident and successful.

At home, Jackson hid an obsession with the rock group Blondie. His memorabilia collection had begun to overflow from his two spare rooms into the entire house. Jackson had spent years buying Blondie items at auctions and online, including T-shirts, ticket stubs, albums and CDs, DVDs, posters, pins, and signed prints.

Blondie represented a time for him when he was young, carefree, and happy. But in his attempt to hang on to that time of his life, his mania had taken over his spare time and space. He was living in the past, and wasn't free to explore happiness in the present.

Like many hoarder collectors, Jackson rationalized that there was real value in this memorabilia aside from its emotional value. But it is rarely the real value of the stuff that makes collectors flip into hoarders.

Most famously, William Randolph Hearst was a hoarder obsessed with collectibles. Certainly his vast collections of art, antiques, and furniture that filled his beautiful mansion in San Simeon, California, were valuable. But he collected so much that the overflow went into storage, never to be seen again after he purchased it. Today San Simeon is a museum, with so much to see in the rotating exhibitions that there are five different tours.

▶ The Food Saver

Janelle had a kitchen full of cans that were twenty years old. She guessed that her refrigerator hadn't been opened in sixteen years—there was too much clutter stacked up in front of it. As soon as we cracked it open, two of my workers started vomiting.

The bins and drawers were full of dark liquid and two inches of green black muck that had once been lettuce. We found black eggs, which at first we thought were carved stone eggs. The food was so moldy that it had all grown together into one gnarly mess.

On the pantry shelves, a lot of the cans were empty. When we looked at them closely we discovered holes gnawed in the bottom. (Rats can get into a can, and once they're in, they'll clean it out. And because they'll stay in a house until there's no food left, Janelle, like most food hoarders, had a severe vermin problem.)

In her mid-sixties, Janelle had raised a family of five boys, all of whom had long since grown and moved away. Her husband had died several years ago, but Janelle was still shopping for bulk food bargains. Her habit continued to spiral out of control, even after her kitchen became all but unusable because of the clutter.

Food hoarders are some of the most reluctant to admit they have a problem. They are often very defensive, arguing that it's not a big deal. Maybe that's because everyone eats, so a food hoarder seems to be collecting something "sensible" that anyone would want.

Food hoarding is exacerbated because hoarders are big on buying food very close to or past its expiration date. Their excuse is that marketers just make up those dates to get customers to buy more food. Even when the cans on Janelle's shelf were bulging, she sometimes ate the contents anyway because she figured the food was safe after it had been cooked. Not surprisingly, her sons were becoming increasingly worried about her health.

The more I work with food hoarders, the more I think their problem may come from a mentality that has something to do with "beating the system." Janelle, for example, took pride in her individuality, and valued her independence. Ignoring food expiration dates was an easy way for her to rebel against authority.

Food hoarders are in hard-core denial, although when confronted they tend to be more embarrassed than pack-rat hoarders because food hoarding is just so messy. Interestingly, it has been my observation that food hoarding prompts more family fights than any other kind.

▶ **The Clothes Hoarder**

Nika is typical of a major subset of hoarders—she couldn't get rid of any clothes. She was a carefully groomed, forty-five-year-old plus-size woman whose weight had fluctuated pretty regularly as she yo-yoed on and off various diets. When she was heavy, she kept her "skinny" clothes because she was convinced that she would lose weight. When she was lighter, she stored her "fat" clothes—just in case. She kept really old clothes because she thought they might come back into style. She even had a cache of clothes, many of which were barely used or even unworn, because she was planning to donate them to charity—when she got around to it.

Nika had clothes stored in the bathroom, where the shower curtain rod had long ago turned the tub into an extra closet. She had so many shoes that they were stored in every room, *in their original boxes*. She had a collection of more than five hundred purses that she couldn't even get to because they were all buried under bags of clothes. In fact, what Nika had was the Great Wall of Clothes, stacked so high and so solidly that it would have held up the ceiling if the house's support beams ever gave out.

For Nika, having a house full of stuff meant she had "made it." Her husband, Andre, didn't agree. And even though the two lived together, Nika admitted that they barely talked. Her hoarding had all but driven him away.

Like many clothes hoarders, Nika had also fallen victim to television home shopping shows, buying the same item in many colors or sizes "just in case" she ran out. The UPS man knew her by name, and even arrived to deliver more packages during Nika's cleaning.

The predatory behaviors of these home shopping networks make it difficult for hoarders to avoid making purchases. The sales techniques target compulsive shoppers in the most insidious ways. For example, they call viewers "friends" and invite them to take advantage of special "insider" opportunities, which appeals to an isolated hoarder's need for friendship and connection. Hoarders like Nika make a choice to buy things, and they are responsible for their actions, but television shopping tactics create a particular challenge that's hard to overcome.

▶ The Memory Keeper

Roxanne lived alone in a trailer home, spending most of her day in dirty sweat suits, sitting in a recliner and chain smoking. She wore her brown hair in a long braid down her back. Her skin was sallow from a liver ailment, and she coughed constantly. Roxanne's adult daughter hadn't been to visit in almost a decade. Roxanne was completely alone—no family, no friends, and no close neighbors. Roxanne didn't have any real relationships, but she did have lots of reminders of her past: She had saved almost every item from her daughter's childhood.

There were two rooms filled five feet high with her daughter's dolls, toys, crafts, and clothes. Roxanne had strollers, a crib, and other old baby equipment that she was convinced her daughter might use one day for her own kids. Roxanne kept saying that her daughter was coming back to pick her things up, but the truth was that her daughter wasn't coming back. In fact, her daughter told us that she'd been happy when she was finally able to move out of that cluttered house and was so fed up with her mother's hoarding that she hadn't returned in ten years.

Hoarders who focus on toys and other childhood possessions are caught up in the past, either their children's or their own, or both. This can spill over into shopping hoarding, but these hoarders aren't buying for themselves; rather, their shopping is usually in an attempt to create memories by buying lots of baby clothes or toddler games for a nephew or grandchild. Curiously, much of what they end up buying is not age-appropriate, in what seems to be an unconscious effort to stop time. And, as in the case of Marcie, the shopaholic, many of the gifts never actually make it to the children but end up added to the piles.

▶ The Trash Master Compactor

Although Margaret is primarily an animal hoarder, she also hoarded trash. She was so overwhelmed that she never got around to taking all the junk to the dump. (Living as she did in a rural community, there was no regular trash pickup even if she'd had the wherewithal to get garbage to the curb.) Instead, the bags piled up around the house or got tossed out into the backyard. For longer than one cared to imagine, food wrappers and a lot of the other trash had just been tossed on the floor and walked on until it became a thick layer of sticky brown muck.

Margaret never consciously decided to save trash. She just fell behind in dealing with it—then got to the point where she gave up caring. Trash hoarding is usually a side effect of hoarding something else.

Information hoarders like Rick can also look like they are hoarding trash, because much of what they hang on to is junk mail or old newspapers. But to Rick, those items have value. Also, hoarders often keep items like paper towel tubes or plastic bags to donate or recycle, and big collections of these can look like trash to non-hoarders.

As we've discovered before, a trash hoarder's piles are as revealing as an archaeological dig. At the bottom are the possessions that may at one time have had some value: clothing, books, toys, household items, and collectibles. Then there are the junk mail, old magazines, and other printed papers that date the point when the hoarder gave up. The top layer is just trash of every sort.

Where Hoarders Hoard

JIM WAS A preacher who started out storing family heir-looms and church artifacts in the garage. He saved boxes of old photographs, knickknacks, and other family items that he felt someone would want someday. He also kept years' worth of church bulletins, linens, and discarded ser-vice accessories like candles and offering plates. He even had an original copy of *Playboy*, which may seem strange for a preacher, but maybe he thought it was a collector's item that would have future value.

After Jim filled up the garage, the collection began to creep into the house. First he filled up the utility room, then the family room. And when Jim's wife died, he filled up the house. We never met Jim, only his children. They organized a cleanup of the house after Jim died.

Hoarding is partly about what the hoarder is collecting, but also sometimes about where. People may not recog-nize a hoarder who has a clean house because they don't see the attic or garage filled to capacity. The hoarder who has the space—the attic, basement, garage, and out-buildings—can stave off the consequences of his or her hoarding for a long time. But eventually the creep takes over and starts invading the hoarder's living space

Once the garage is filled, of course, many hoarders have to park their cars outside. And for many, a car is just another place to store stuff. In the next chapter, we'll meet Ben, the pizza man, whose car was filled with so many empty pizza boxes—and had become so disgusting—that he had to buy another car to get around.

Backyard junkyards (or in some cases, front-yard junk-yards) are popular hoarding locations. This is where you'll

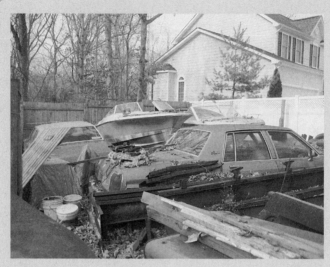

Much to the consternation of their neighbors, property values go down when hoarders spread to the outdoors and the piles mount.

find the big stuff—old appliances, cars, lawn care equipment, furniture (outdoor and indoor). Often the backyard hoarder will claim that the value of the scrap metal makes it worth keeping lots of this stuff. I once found an entire barn filled with aluminum cans, probably worth about $10,000. We didn't cash them in because we ran out of time on the cleanup. That hoarder is still working on taking his cans to the recycling facility, one bag at a time.

Outside hoarding is dangerous—and in most cases unlawful. Not only does it attract snakes, rats, mosquitoes (to standing water), and noxious weeds, it also attracts the attention of local authorities. Yard hoarders are often the first to be cited and fined since junked cars and appliances that contain gas, Freon, or other high-risk materials are significant health hazards. A hoarder with lots of land can seemingly keep collecting forever because there are no ceilings or walls outside.

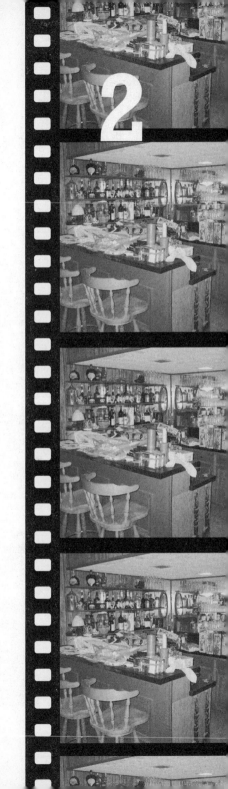

WHY
PEOPLE
HOARD

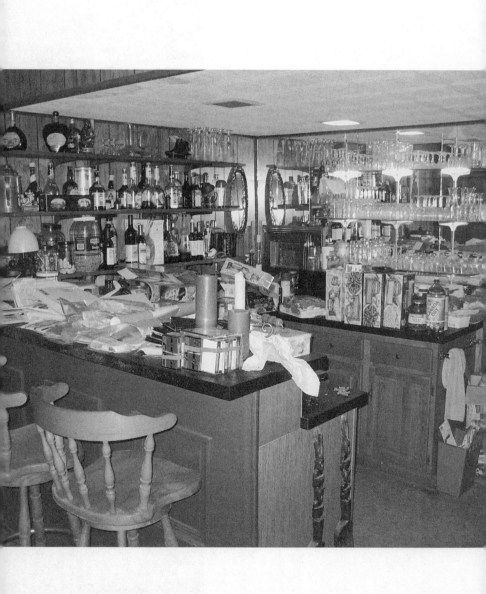

At just over six feet tall, with long blond hair, Candace, fifty-nine, was an imposing figure. She had been a well-paid advertising executive who had also taught classes on marketing at the university near her upscale neighborhood. She confided that money wasn't an issue for her as she'd invested well and was able to retire from both her advertising job and teaching.

But years before Clutter Cleaner came into her life, Candace had slipped into horrible living conditions. In her house, my crew and I were faced with heaps of papers, clothes, books, and trash in every room, all but burying what I came to discover was a lot of fine antique furniture. One bedroom was so completely filled with junk that the door would barely open. Extension cords crisscrossed the rooms because the electrical outlets had been blocked ages ago. And the whole house reeked of dog feces and urine.

Candace hadn't been a lifelong hoarder, but a difficult divorce followed immediately by her mother's death sent her into a tailspin. She started drinking heavily—and the years of self-abuse were starting to show on her face—and in the way she lived.

Her mother had left everything to Candace, who took her mother's possessions into her own home but hadn't bothered to sort, give away, or discard anything.

And the more she drank, the less she cared about keeping

a clean house. She started to fall behind on simple daily tasks like sorting through mail, taking the dogs out, or getting rid of old clothes. As a person who had been used to being on top of everything, she felt her frustration turn into depression and exacerbate what was already becoming an untenable living situation.

There were clear signs that Candace had obsessive-compulsive tendencies. Under the piles of things in her house were shelves and storage bins that had been put into place at one time to control clutter. Her framed pictures and other knickknacks were neatly labeled with notes on the back or underneath explaining what they were and who they came from. Her dresser drawers were marked "darks" and "whites" for her clothes.

Even her squalor was OCD. Although the dogs were going to the bathroom in the house, Candace had limited them to two rooms. Her piles were organized into categories—books, clothes, papers. The house was a mess, and whatever earlier attempts she had made to stay in control had been all but abandoned.

Candace admitted that once she fell behind on her organization, she *really* fell behind. She couldn't accept the middle ground of mild, occasional clutter that most people live in. For Candace, everything was black or white, just like the labels for her clothing. A house that had once been so precisely organized and labeled was now an out-and-out disaster area. She had simply given up the struggle.

Like almost every hoarder with whom I've worked, Candace also showed signs of what I now know to be clinical depression: She didn't smile or make eye contact; her voice was flat, without any affect. She admitted that she had trouble getting out of bed in the morning and struggled to make simple decisions.

Candace was clearly an intelligent woman. At one time she had enjoyed spending time with her family and friends, but her social life had tapered off years ago. She seemed to have made a choice: A house full of clutter with its piles of clothes, books, and papers was more important than living what would be by most people's standards a normal life that included family and friends, hobbies and pastimes, entertainment and travel.

Those frustrated family and friends, who mostly find themselves excluded from a hoarder's life, may wonder why their loved one can't just throw away those ten years' worth of newspapers piled up in the garage, the piles of old and never-before-worn clothes, or the junk that seems to grow organically in every corner. Wouldn't a sane person just recycle, toss, or give away this stuff—and move on?

But while a hoarder may not be certifiable, his or her brain does work differently. Hoarding specialist Dr. Renae Reinardy often compares hoarders to parents with dyslexia who wish to read bedtime stories to their children, but no matter how desperately they want to do it, their brains simply will not cooperate.

I'm not a psychologist or a psychiatrist, although I do work alongside therapists and other health care professionals with many of my clients. But one learns a lot about a person in such intimate circumstances as a cleanup. I've found that it is important not only to help the hoarders get rid of stuff, but also to really talk with them—swapping stories and sharing experiences as we do the cleaning. The issues, both physical and psychological, they are wrestling with quickly become clear during this process.

I've learned that most hoarders love their families deeply and long to reestablish lost or strained relationships. Hoarders are truly in pain from losing their connection with loved ones—and the world at large. Ironically, the only way they see to ease that pain is to literally and figuratively bury themselves more deeply.

The more time I spend with hoarders, the more I wonder

THE SECRET LIVES OF HOARDERS

what propels them down this path. Everyone has issues. Bad things happen. The clues to why people hoard are not so simple or straightforward to decipher but may be discovered in the complex interaction of personality and circumstances, in an individual's ability to respond to life events in a certain way, in genetics, or in more serious psychiatric issues that manifest themselves in classic hoarding behavior.

IT'S ALL IN THE FAMILY

One thing that has become fairly obvious to me when I work with clients and their families is the likelihood that the hoarder is not the only one with an issue. As with other medical and psychological conditions, there's much discussion concerning the genetic roots of hoarding. And if my experiences and observations have shown me anything, it's that hoarding—like blue eyes or curly hair—can be a family trait.

One of my clients, Pat, had the help of her mother during her cleanup. Pat and her mother, who were both overweight and wore similar sweat suits with lots of gold jewelry, looked more like sisters than mother and daughter. They even bickered like sisters. Every time Pat chose an item to donate or throw away, her mother would move in and say something like, "That's nice, maybe we should keep that." By the end of the first day, Pat's mother had loaded her own car and had even more of Pat's castoffs in a pile by the front door. Pat told me that her mother's hoarding problem was even worse than her own, which is something I hear all the time: "If you think this is bad, you should see my mother/grandfather/aunt!"

A report published in *Behavior Research and Therapy* found that hoarding appears to run in some families where OCD is also present. And a study done at the Obsessive-Compulsive Disorders Clinic at the University of California in 2009 found that up to 85 percent of people who are compulsive hoarders have a close relative who is or was also a hoarder. A Johns Hopkins study found significant linkage to compulsive hoarding on chromosome 14 in families with obsessive-compulsive disorder.

It's not surprising that as I've dug into my clients' backgrounds I've discovered a pattern of hoarding along with other family traits.

TRIGGERS

While there are clearly links to other mental disorders, several of which I'll discuss later in this chapter, from my observations it seems that every hoarder has had an event, or series of events, that either marked the start of that person's hoarding or made an already established hoarding habit much worse.

All of us face challenges in life. Divorce, death, job loss, relationship breakups, or medical issues—those are some of the hardest things anyone can go through. For hoarders, there are many common themes, the most compelling of which is abuse.

Roxanne, who had kept all of her grown daughter's stuff from the time she was an infant, is a not uncommon case. As Roxanne and I worked through cleaning out her spare rooms, she shared with me that she had been abused as a child. Roxanne realized that by saving her daughter's things, she felt like she was preserving and protecting her daughter's childhood. She was really trying to find a childhood that she never had. She didn't understand that hoarding her daughter's possessions had actually pushed her daughter out of her life.

I've seen hoarders whose habit was triggered by events as wide-ranging as a cheating boyfriend or a diagnosis of cancer. One client had lost a child in a car accident and then two weeks later her husband died. Another started hoarding after her husband shot himself in the backyard. Sometimes a hoarder is so deep in depression that the story takes on facets that probably never even happened, but the hoarder believes that they did. I call those "false triggers." True or false, the triggers are real in the hoarder's mind.

There always seems to be an emotional event that triggers the behavior. Finding that is the job of the therapist and the hoarder. But family members and those who work with a hoarder need to understand that collecting things is what hoarders frequently do to comfort themselves after trauma. Anyone coming in to clean is coming in to take away those comfort items. That makes the cleanup person a real threat, even if the hoarder is asking for help.

Almost every hoarder I've worked with has experienced tragedy. They are sad and feel alone and isolated. Hoarders do not consciously choose to live the way they do; it's a defensive reaction to what happened or what they believe happened. Family members and professionals can help by remembering that there is a cause, instead of focusing solely on getting rid of the trash.

The triggers never go away: They are life-changing traumas that will always cause some pain. The memories come up often, unexpectedly, and usually when someone is already under stress. Or a hoarder may not even be aware of the trigger, and so it happens in the subconscious. In response, hoarders turn to their possessions, maybe shopping to add to the hoard, or retreating to be with their pets, or creating more piles.

Becoming a hoarder is not unlike becoming a workaholic or an exercise fanatic as a way to escape a difficult life or event. People can turn to these activities just like hoarders rely on acquiring and holding on to their stuff. Work can be a place where someone can feel safe and confident. Exercise can be an activity that makes someone feel better. But anything taken to extremes will inevitably become a problem. In an ideal world, the hoarder would learn to recognize triggers and then respond with a healthier, more balanced behavior that's equally comforting. But that's usually a task best undertaken with a counselor, not a cleaner.

Not all hoarders figure out their triggers, but Marcie, the shopaholic, was able to do so. As we worked on cleaning her house, Marcie started talking about why she shopped so much and saved it all, and she confessed that she wanted to figure out what had made her become this person.

In our time together, I had noticed that her husband was a big, angry guy. He yelled at her a lot during the cleanup, and I wondered if it went further than yelling. I mentioned the yelling to Marcie, and she was pretty frank in asking me if it was obvious that he hit her. She kept talking about it, wondering if she was hanging on to things to comfort herself, to feel safe and protected.

I've witnessed cases like Marcie's repeatedly. Hoarders aren't slobs who don't care about being clean. They are people struggling with overwhelming emotional issues. A pile in a hoarder house isn't a pile of stuff; it can be many things: a pile of sadness, a pile of quitting, or sometimes even a pile of hope. It's never really about the stuff, hoarders are just confusing their possessions with their emotions.

BOUNDARIES

Regardless of what triggers a person to turn to hoarding, there is one characteristic that I have found to be pretty common to all of the people with whom I've worked: They struggle with limits and boundaries. Margaret, for example, loved her animals because they made her happy. One dog, or maybe even three, would have been manageable for her. But she wasn't able to put that limit on herself. In Margaret's mind, if one dog made her happy, a hundred dogs would make her a hundred times happier. Putting a limit on how many dogs she could accept into her household would be like putting a limit on her happiness, and she wasn't willing to do that.

For hoarders who shop (or Dumpster dive), it's the same issue. Purchasing an item gives them a rush of temporary joy, so purchasing more items seems like it should give them an even bigger rush. The collecting gets out of hand when hoarders become so compulsive that they can't limit it. It's also a problem when hoarding is the only thing that brings the person happiness, instead of family, friendships, hobbies, work, exercise, or other pastimes.

Dr. Suzanne Chabaud, who works with OCD patients and hoarders at her clinic in New Orleans, points out that hoarders need to learn to have appropriate boundaries. A shopping hoarder may be buying lots of items ostensibly for her husband and her children, but in actuality they don't want them. The shopaholic isn't respecting their boundaries. She is focused on what *she* wants for them instead of what they actually want—or need from her.

Conversely, hoarders may put limits into place that aren't appropriate, such as when they don't let people come into their lives to help or simply to form friendships. These limits, like the hoarding itself, may be in response to the imagined and unnamed fears and threats that plague the hoarder's life.

AVOIDING REALITY

Whatever the triggers that set off the hoarding may be, or whatever boundaries and limits with which the hoarders wrestle, almost every person I've worked with has been fixated either on the future or the past. It's so much easier than living in the present, because the present can be awfully depressing. Since the present is clouded by strained family relationships, financial and personal challenges as well as the clutter, it's very tempting for hoarders to avoid the realities completely and focus instead on a fantasy. Hoarders also look for an escape into what I call "easy love," and this is particularly true with animal hoarders. Whatever they are collecting, hoarders turn to their things or pets for positive reinforcement, because that's a lot less complicated than trying to have a rewarding relationship with another person.

▶ Fake Future

Ben, who we introduced earlier in the book as the "pizza man," had a house and car crammed with old pizza boxes. In addition, he had a basement full of bits and pieces of mechanical airplane parts, which Ben claimed were enough to build three complete airplanes. To hear him tell it, these would be vintage, collectible airplanes from the golden age of aviation, and he just knew that he was going to build those airplanes and sell them to a museum. In his mind's eye, he saw himself becoming a sought-after expert on cloth-wing biplanes. He would write a book and appear on television, giving commentary on aircraft building and restoration. Maybe he would even get a job at the Smithsonian Air and Space Museum, which was near where he lived.

The dream was all Ben talked about. It was so much more appealing than the reality of living in a dangerously full, Stage 5 hoarded house that was getting worse day by day. Ben saw only the fantasy of his completed airplanes, not the thousands of unassembled parts or the putrid rotting pizza that was decaying on top of them. Ben didn't see himself as an out-of-control hoarder—he was a man with a plan. Unfortunately, Ben wasn't taking any steps toward implementing that plan. His brain had completely skipped over the phase of picking up the tools, clearing a work space, and starting to assemble the parts of the plane. Instead, Ben was living entirely in the "reward" phase, giving himself lots of praise for being an aviation expert in the making. In his mind, he was happily on his way toward that inevitable, wonderful future.

The reality for Ben was that getting rid of his clutter might have cleared enough space for him to start a few actual projects. But in his mind, throwing *anything* away was tantamount to throwing away that glittering future. In his mind he simply couldn't separate the junk from the valuables—or wasn't prepared to cope with the task of separating one from the other.

For hoarders, the fake future is the place where they will be successful and happy, and everyone will love them. They can't think about what others close to them may want—or need—such as a clean house or more quality time together. To make a significant change in their lives, hoarders like Ben or Lucy, the crafter, have to reject their fantasies and learn to accept whatever rewards of reality they can.

▶ Perfect Past

Roxanne was hoarding her daughter's baby items to hold on to a past that never really existed. Her relationship with her daughter had always been strained, and since the daughter had moved out she had broken off all contact with Roxanne. That separation was too painful for Roxanne, so she spent ten years building an alternative reality.

Roxanne's thoughts of the past were colored with nostalgia for a time when there were no arguments, no blame, and no hoarding. Each doll or teddy bear conjured up feel-good memories. As long as she had the mementos, she could visit that fantasyland anytime she wanted to escape the bleak reality of her trailer park home, her isolation, and her deteriorating health.

It has been my experience that many hoarders, like Roxanne, are trying to cope with a tragic childhood. And they have to take a huge and very painful leap into reality each time they agree to part with a possession.

▶ **Easy Love**

For a hoarder like Margaret, animals are a source of unconditional love. They are always around for a pat or a hug, they are always happy to see her, and they won't voluntarily leave. It's an easy relationship for her to maintain—she feeds and pets them, and they love her unconditionally. They don't demand anything, they don't offer any challenges, and most importantly, they don't complain about the hoarding.

I have worked with many hoarders who have had failed relationships, often through no fault of their own. Many were abused as children or have been in abusive marriages. Someone who has been hurt that badly has trouble trusting again. Instead, attaching to animals or possessions is much safer and easier. When given the opportunity to get another pet, animal hoarders focus on that easy love and not the reality of whether or not they can actually take care of the animal.

Ironically, the hoarding also keeps people at bay—people hoarders see as threatening. Safe behind the piles, where nobody will reach out and try to engage them in a healthy relationship, hoarders don't run the risk of being hurt again. Taking hoarders' stuff makes them feel vulnerable; they lose their safety net, and that's a terrifying prospect.

THE HOARDER'S STATE OF MIND

To the outsider, the hoarder may appear to be lazy, hostile, or irrational. But really, it's about deep-seated sadness or anger that may mask or be exacerbated by other mental disorders.

I didn't set out to write a medical textbook but rather to dispel some of the myths that surround hoarding and give those who are trying to help a sense of the underlying causes of this condition. For family, friends, and professionals whose response may go quickly from sympathy to exasperation and resentment, it is helpful to have an understanding of the psychology of the hoarder—and all the factors that play into this pathology.

Over the years on the front lines, I've worked closely with mental health professionals and read whatever I could find on the clinical research. (For a good overview of what's been published, see the resources listed at the end of the book.)

However, even research psychologists aren't sure exactly what's going on. They do know that hoarding is not simply laziness. It is not confined to the poor and undereducated. It is most definitely a psychological disorder. But, like so many disorders, it may be described as a syndrome that is manifested in any number of behaviors.

Researchers also know that hoarders often have other identifiable medical issues, including dementia, obsessive-compulsive disorder, and depression. But they're still figuring out if the other diseases lead to hoarding or if hoarding triggers them. And it's not clear whether hoarding is its own mental disorder or a subset of some other category.

Dr. Suzanne Chabaud explains that researchers are discovering that although hoarding is being recognized as a symptom of certain disorders, like dementia and schizophrenia, there are other cases in which they are questioning the connection. For example, do hoarders with depression, anxiety, or attention deficit/hyperactivity disorder (ADHD) hoard because of those disorders, or do they develop those disorders separate from hoarding? Called "co-morbid disorders," they often develop in tandem, but without clear proof showing that one causes the other.

In my work, I have almost always found there to be another definable mental disorder in evidence. When therapists or counselors like Dr. Chabaud work with hoarders, they try to find out what that other disorder (or disorders) might be, since simply getting a hoarder's place cleaned up doesn't address the underlying causes that led to the problem in the first place. The work doesn't end when the dump truck pulls away from the house. The real work is just getting started.

I don't play therapist with my clients. I am more of a coach, who also gets involved in the heavy lifting and logistics. But once my part of the job is complete, I want to know that I've done everything I can to set these folks on the path to recovery. Understanding the range of conditions that drive or accompany hoarding helps me to do that—and will be invaluable to anyone in this situation.

▶ Obsessive-Compulsive Disorder

Candace, whose story opened this chapter, had been in therapy and was diagnosed with obsessive-compulsive disorder (OCD). She's not unusual—hoarding has traditionally been linked to OCD. One research study at Johns Hopkins found that up to 42 percent of patients with OCD were also hoarders.

At first glance this doesn't make much sense. People with OCD are stereotyped as being off-the-charts clean and tidy, with all kinds of rules about items not touching each other and everything being in its special place. That doesn't sound like hoarding.

Ironically, that obsession is actually the root of the problem. Candace frequently got bogged down while she was trying to get control of her stuff because she couldn't make the *perfect* decision about what to do with her things. This dilemma created a constant internal struggle.

Candace would look at a stack of books and want to line them up neatly on a shelf. But of course there was no empty shelf in her house. Based on her behavior during the initial stages of the cleanup, I can only imagine her internal dialogue: "You're doing this all wrong, you need an empty shelf. Don't listen to those people trying to help you; they don't know how to do it correctly. You can do the job way better by yourself. There's just so much to do besides these books, and wait, you are doing it all wrong!"

So instead of cleaning off a shelf, or maybe deciding to donate the books, Candace became overwhelmed and exhausted and would then just toss the books onto a growing pile. She truly believed she would get to the mess later, but later never came.

Obsessive people can also become overwhelmed by fears: of losing an important item or information; of others touching or moving their possessions; of missing out on a special sale purchase. The sum of these fears can contribute to hoarding. Just as a person with classic OCD finds relief in repetitious actions or rituals, some OCD hoarders collect things not only to feel good but also to fight off discomfort and pain. Dr. Chabaud has worked with OCD hoarders who are driven by a need to protect their families—they feel if they don't buy a spare set of sheets then their entire family will be in peril because a hurricane might come one day and level the house, and leave them with no bedding.

There are a few other classic yet rarer OCD symptoms that can lead to hoarding. A person with an obsession for cleanliness won't touch anything that has touched the floor. So whatever falls there remains there—and accumulates exponentially. Some people develop a compulsion to save hair or nail clippings, feces, or anything they may have touched, and they won't get rid of it. There can be process compulsions—the need to go through a long mental checklist before an item can be thrown away. Rather than go through this ritual, the hoarder will postpone the decision and the stuff piles up. I've also heard of OCD hoarders who become obsessed with buying sets of things, or buying things in even numbers.

When hoarding is driven by OCD, it's all about perfectionism, indecision, and procrastination. You will see the hoarder get bogged down in making decisions about which items to donate, throw away, or keep. He or she will probably have to touch every item as it leaves the house, checking things off on a "mental inventory." A hoarder with OCD can often handle the items leaving a home, but not knowing if the item is there or not messes up the inventory in his or her head and creates constant mental violence.

Children Who Hoard

DR. SUZANNE CHABAUD, who works with clients with OCD and hoarding issues, says a significant number of children with OCD are also hoarders and their hoarding is sometimes a very early symptom. Kids who hoard have a lower response to medication than OCD kids who don't hoard.

Hoarder children exhibit pronounced tendencies of indecision, procrastination, and perfectionism. They don't want to let things go, they can't make a choice about what toys to keep and what to donate. Or the children get fixated on "just right." For instance, they find the exactly perfect place for a stuffed bear, and then the bear can't be moved. Moving the bear would upset the perfect order of things.

Not all children who become hoarders have OCD, of course. Their behavior may be learned if they are growing up in a hoarder house. Some children of hoarders never learn to set limits on their possessions, or basic cleaning and organizing techniques. On the other hand, children with OCD may react in exactly the opposite way, and always try to carve out a neat little space for themselves in a cluttered household.

▶ Anxiety

With her long denim jumper, huge blue eyes, and helmet of gray hair, Thalia looked every inch the kindly grandmother that she was. Thalia was also a Stage 5 hoarder whose incessant talking and constant fluttering of her hands were classic signs of high anxiety. Time and again during her cleanup, she became so agitated that she would suffer a meltdown and the entire process would come to a halt. She admitted that she was in therapy, and she had prescription medication bottles littered through the house. But if any of it was anti-anxiety medication, it didn't seem to be very effective.

Thalia's house was full of knickknacks like salt and pepper shakers and other china figurines. She also had lots of memorabilia from her volunteer work in local elections in her Pennsylvania suburb—banners, yard signs, photos of her with the candidates.

Thalia's anxiety was so high that she was unable to make any decision—ever. A stack of campaign flyers would send her into a tizzy. One can only imagine what was going on in her head:

What if there is something important in that stack of documents and it gets thrown away? What if one of these flyers is valuable because it is now history? Is all this memorabilia worth any money? Could anyone I care about use that flyer? Will my family finally love me because I saved them these valuable historical documents? Wait, there may be some cockroaches in those papers, maybe they are too gross to move. I don't want to make a mess because then I will have to clean up. Who would I call to take care of the roaches? Can I afford to hire pest control? Oh no, I don't want anyone to see my house. Wow, what time is it? I really need to get working on these papers. But now I'm tired, I'll lie down and rest. I'll worry about the papers tomorrow. What do I have to do tomorrow? Do I have anything important I have forgotten? Where is my phone? Oh no, I can't find my phone. Did I lose my cell phone or did someone steal it? I bet someone stole my cell phone. Oh no, I can't afford a new phone. What am I going to do . . . ? Oh, here it is under some papers. Gosh, there sure is a lot of paper here. What am I going to do about all this paper? I wonder if there is something important in these papers. . . .

Anxiety can completely paralyze a hoarder. Thalia was simply unable to help herself. Even though she wasn't physically active, her mental gymnastics exhausted her. When anxiety becomes this crippling, it needs to be treated with medication and/or therapy before cleaning can even begin.

Anxiety disorder is a general term that covers a range conditions including panic disorder, several phobias, obsessive-compulsive disorder, and post-traumatic stress disorder. (OCD hoarders have traditionally been grouped under anxiety disorder, but they have been discussed separately since they do portray distinctive behavioral characteristics.)

The latest studies on hoarding suggest that it may be its own subset of anxiety disorder and not part of OCD. Researchers are debating whether there should be a new category of psychology called "compulsive disorders," which would include hoarding, OCD, and perhaps drug and alcohol abuse.

While the medical profession is still figuring out how all of these disorders are connected, in my experience, most hoarders have anxiety issues. Dr. Chabaud points out that a hoarder's intense apprehensiveness is driven by fear—fear of real or imagined danger. All hoarders are attached to their objects, and so all of them will get anxious when someone starts taking those items away. A hoarder who has spent twenty years collecting something begins to identify with those items. Taking them away is like taking *the person* away. Anxiety is a natural reaction to such a severe threat.

Dr. Chabaud also says that hoarders who have a compulsive need to shop, for example, do so because it reduces their anxiety. The urge to buy is so intense that if someone tells the hoarder to stop, he or she starts to feel angry, irritable, scared, and anxious. People often ask me how a hoarder can have the energy to shop, but not have the energy to clean. For a hoarder, shopping has nothing to do with energy; it is completely about relieving anxiety and feeling good.

Hoarders are quick to go into anxiety mode when faced with making a decision about throwing items away. The anxiety is so overwhelming, and painful, that the hoarder avoids it by postponing decisions. Hoarders truly believe that they will get to the task tomorrow, but that day never comes.

▶ Attention Deficit (Hyperactivity) Disorder (ADD/ADHD)

Lucy, the craft hoarder who baked all the cakes, wanted to finally clean out her house after she retired. As long as someone was there working alongside Lucy, she was on it. She was hyper-focused on cleaning, and she could get through a room more quickly than most hoarders I've worked with. But on the days that nobody was helping her, and she had boxes to sort through on her own, she got too distracted to do the job. Unfortunately, she would go shopping instead.

Lucy would go shopping and load up on craft items, not stopping to think about the reality of what she really had time to do. "I can crochet a hundred fifty baby blankets this year," she would tell herself. "I know I only made three last year, but this year will be different. I have to buy all this yarn now so I can have my materials on hand when I'm ready to get started. If I go ahead and buy the yarn, then that will motivate me to actually get it done! And these cookie sheets are on sale; if I buy them, I will finish the blankets faster since I also want to make cookies. I know! I'll give cookies along with the blankets! I just have to stay focused and I can totally do it."

Lucy's ADHD drove her hoarding in that she was distracted by too many hobbies and bought endless supplies for each one. Also, she didn't keep track of what she already had, so she was buying duplicates.

Lucy was smart, and she wanted to stay clean. This wasn't about laziness or a lack of education. Lucy's brain just worked differently. Hoarders like her have got to treat the ADHD first, usually with a combination of medication and therapy, or they just won't be able to master the processes required to stay clutter-free.

The connection to ADHD is an easy one to make. Someone who is easily distracted and has difficulty sticking to a plan could become overwhelmed by keeping track of his or her possessions.

Dr. Chabaud has found that with ADHD, it's difficult to tell which comes first. For example, do people start hoarding because they have ADHD issues, can't focus, and over-buy when shopping? Or is it that a hoarder is so confused by the collecting compulsion that his or her brain starts to get easily distracted in other areas?

Because Lucy was easily distracted, she just wasn't going to reliably follow through with things like folding laundry, washing dirty dishes, or even getting basic housekeeping done. And once she fell behind on those tasks, she felt so overwhelmed that she had no idea where to even start.

The hallmark of ADHD is that the "executive function" part of the brain doesn't work very well. This is the brain's "boss," essentially, driving the person's ability to sort, prioritize, and categorize tasks. A hoarder with ADHD can't really make rational decisions about what to do. This hoarder also tends to fight structure and order, preferring to be spontaneous. Organization can look too controlling to a person with ADHD, like it might stifle the person's creativity and impetuous nature.

Throwing items away seems risky, because in the ADHD world things are always getting misplaced. If an item with sentimental value gets lost, the memories might disappear with it, so the hoarder prefers to just keep everything. The most important items—whatever the ADHD person is holding at the moment—go "right here on top" of the piles. That's how the piles grow. Everything in every pile is in some way important to a hoarder.

Also, ADHD hoarders have trouble thinking through "what-if" scenarios. For example, how likely is the hoarder to actually fix that broken clock radio? What are the chances the hoarder will actually find the missing pieces to the board game? More important, with whom is the hoarder going to play that game? These scenarios probably aren't going to end satisfactorily, but someone with impaired executive function in the brain can't weigh the likelihood of that.

Finally, another hallmark of ADHD is the tendency to *overfocus* on a process or event and lose sight of the big picture, which means Lucy may not have even seen the house in its entirety. She may have seen only one pile at a time, and not realized—or subconsciously chosen not to accept—the extent of the problem.

▶ Addiction

Kurt was a shopping hoarder whose house, like Marcie's, was filled with purchases still in their original bags and packaging. He was a compulsive shopper who lived for the thrill of finding a sale item, of comparing pricing and getting value for his money. Kurt liked nothing better than to deck himself out in a suit, gold chains, and watch; spritz on a little cologne; style his toupee—and go shopping. He felt important and totally in control.

Kurt admitted that he knew he was getting himself into debt and worsening his hoarding, but the act of shopping made him feel so good that he justified it to himself. On any given day he'd head off to his favorite big-box store, and he might tell himself that he'd just see what the sales were but wouldn't actually buy anything. But then he would come home with hundreds of dollars' worth of items. One could imagine his rationalization: "I know I shouldn't do this; my credit card is maxed out. But this jacket fits me perfectly and it's such a bargain. And my sister would love this silk flower arrangement. If I buy it for her, then she will come over and we can sit and have coffee like we used to. I should get new coffee mugs since this set is on sale. What the heck, my credit card will probably get turned down anyway."

When Kurt's card went through and he had toted his new purchases home, the guilt would set in. "I shouldn't have bought that much stuff," he would think. "I have got to stop shopping so much. I will bring those mugs back tomorrow. I'll put them on this pile of other things that I have got to take back. Boy, this place is a mess. I have got to start sorting through this stuff and sell some of it online. I know I can get a lot of money for it." But instead of sorting, Kurt would just go shopping again the next day.

According to Dr. Chabaud, researchers are still debating about whether hoarding is an impulse disorder, a compulsion, or an addiction. While one may casually use the term "shopaholic" to describe people like Kurt and Marcie, a true "addiction" would indicate that the addict goes through *physical* withdrawal symptoms if he or she tries to stop the behavior. Anecdotally, I don't see this happening with hoarders. To me their behavior looks more like a compulsion, which is a behavior that feels so good that a person does it to excess. I do see serious hoarding compulsions that have a lot in common with addictions like alcoholism and drug addiction, and I'm not a psychologist, so I tend to use the word "addiction" to describe hoarding, even though it may truly be more of a compulsion.

Hoarders who shop, or who go "Dumpster diving," definitely do it because it feels good. These hoarders get a primal rush from the "hunt and gather" experience. This rush helps them avoid the reality of what is truly going on in their lives. Rescuing a broken television set from someone's alleyway trash pile is a thrill. These hoarders don't stop to think about whether or not they have the time to fix that TV, along with the dozens of other broken appliances they have gathered.

For collectors, the excitement of finding a long-sought, rare Michael Jackson album on vinyl is all about scoring. They're never going to play it. But they feel powerful and happy when they buy it. The hoarder feels like a success because he or she just got a valuable item. There's a level of excitement that releases adrenaline in the brain, and when that adrenaline high fades, the hoarder goes back for more. That's when it begins to look like an addiction, because the hoarder's happiness is linked to the item, not to any sense of self-worth.

Animal hoarders have a similar thing going on, with the constant love they get from their pets. Anytime an animal hoarder feels down, there's a cat right there to share some affection, which can quickly become a substitute for human relationships. Receiving love endorphin hits all day is a happy way for anyone to live. Hoarders get to feel that exciting rush every time they go shopping, go Dumpster diving, or reach for one of three dozen affectionate dogs. Especially when the rest of a hoarder's life isn't going well, it's easy to see how this behavior could become an addiction.

Some experts argue that addicts never change their personalities; they just substitute healthy addictions for unhealthy ones. So a smoker might give up cigarettes and turn instead to the exercise addiction of running marathons. I see this sometimes with hoarders, and I encourage the replacement behavior if it seems positive.

For example, as we cleaned Kurt's house, it became clear that it needed major repairs. The bathrooms had extensive water damage and needed to be redone, the kitchen needed new cabinets and appliances, and the whole downstairs required new walls and flooring. I encouraged Kurt to channel his shopping energy into the remodel. He threw himself into choosing appliances and researching subcontractors. This work kept him focused on making positive decisions. Suddenly, Kurt's shopping had purpose. Luckily, when the remodel was over, Kurt became very involved in his church's upcoming remodel. Although Kurt hasn't had counseling to deal with the real issues behind his hoarding, he has successfully rechanneled that energy into more positive behavior.

I have done this in my own life. I replaced my gambling addiction with work. Some may say I'm just as addicted to cleaning as I was to gambling, and they might be right. For me it worked to substitute a positive addiction for something negative. I haven't gambled since 1999, and I've refocused my life to revolve around my family and my work. I'm not saying that's scientifically or psychologically correct, but for me it worked.

▶ **Depression**

Roxanne, the hoarder who saved all of her daughter's items, showed all the classic signs of depression. She didn't make eye contact or smile when she spoke in a colorless monotone. She wore the same clothes for several weeks in a row, even when they were covered with food stains. Her dirty brown hair was pulled into a messy ponytail, and she admitted that she didn't wash herself regularly. Roxanne ate a lot of fast food, and she was overweight.

When Roxanne opened a package of food, she tossed the wrapper on the floor with a "why bother" attitude. She had basically given up—some days, she just stayed in bed.

Depression is a crippling illness, erasing a person's desire and ability to make daily life decisions. Someone who is depressed usually knows what to do in order to get better but can't muster the energy to actually do it. To a depressed person, even a small job like getting out of bed or taking a shower can look overwhelmingly hopeless and impossible.

A depressed person withdraws from normal life in the same way that a hoarder does. Depression is marked by decreasing interest in organization, self-care, and interaction with the outside world, which are all traits I see often in advanced hoarders.

Depressed people seem to be perpetually sad, angry, or anxious. Eventually, if the disease isn't treated, depressed people can become so frustrated and worn down by their negative outlook that they become suicidal. I've seen this in hoarders too, and it should be taken seriously.

This is another situation where it's not clear which comes first—depression or hoarding. Dr. Chabaud says that depression in someone who is genetically predisposed may be triggered by a traumatic event. That same event can also trigger hoarding behavior, and the two disorders can develop simultaneously.

Ironically, I've noticed that hoarders who are depressed usually don't fight a cleanup. They just lack the initiative to make the push and get it done themselves, and they generally accept help. However, under these circumstances, it is even more important to understand that the cleanup on its own will not solve the problem. Unless the underlying issues are resolved, the hoarding will come back. Depression isn't just an annoyance; it can lead to a seriously life-threatening situation.

▶ Social Phobia

Ben, the "pizza man" who also hoarded vintage airplane parts, was shy and uncomfortable around people. He avoided group settings because they made him anxious. Ben seemed to have an issue that Dr. Chabaud says is sometimes linked with hoarding—social phobia.

Hoarders who have a social disorder connect more with the world of objects than with people. Their possessions become their friends. Those possessions won't threaten them with pressing questions or awkward social moments. Hoarders can control their relationship with these items more than they can control relationships with friends or family members.

This disorder, Dr. Chabaud says, isn't necessarily a symptom of hoarding, or a cause. Like depression, social phobia can show up in hoarders, but it's not clear which disorder came first, or if one triggered the other.

One of the keys to success on a hoarder cleanup is to get the hoarder back into the world and involved in outside activities and a social life. For that reason, any social disorder needs to be treated as part of a hoarder's recovery therapy.

▶ Dementia

Rick, the retired professor with a house full of paper, was showing signs of dementia when the cleanup began. He was very forgetful, often standing in the living room hunched over in confusion and asking the same question over and over. Sometimes he didn't recognize an item he had in his hand, or remember why he was holding it. His sister commented that the problem had been worsening over the past year.

He had focused on information hoarding during a lifetime as a professor, but his forgetfulness had exacerbated the problem. He would pick up something, intending to use it or throw it away, and then forget why he was holding it. Confused, he would just set it down again on a growing pile.

A study published in the *American Journal of Geriatric Psychiatry* found that 23 percent of patients with dementia also showed hoarding behavior. As the population ages, dementia—and hoarding—will increasingly become severe problems, which need to be addressed in tandem. When a hoarder isn't even able to have a coherent conversation about the issue, interventions are essential if the hoarder is living in conditions that are physically dangerous or unhealthy.

WHY GET INVOLVED?

Aside from the emotional toll that hoarding takes, it can make conditions physically unsafe for the hoarder. Piles can fall over and germs can cause illness. A cluttered house can hide serious structural damage. An elderly hoarder can have trouble getting around, and if there are medical issues, it's sometimes impossible for emergency medical teams to even get into the house to respond.

As we have discussed, hoarding is—and often disguises— a severe mental problem, as hoarders tend to be isolated, cutting themselves off, socially and emotionally, even when they crave human interaction. If a hoarder also has a related mental disorder, that often goes untreated.

Hoarding affects more than just a hoarder. Children growing up in a hoarder house don't learn to set limits on their possessions and sometimes on their behavior. I've seen those bad habits spill over into work attitudes and financial management, so that a child of a hoarder struggles to follow rules on the job or stick to a budget. Children of hoarders talk about the emotional trauma of feeling like their hoarder parent chose hoarding over his or her children. And some of them grow up to become hoarders themselves.

Hoarders also make a big financial mess that someone else often has to clean up. Hoarders who spend money on their acquisitions usually end up broke and dependent on family members, or the government, for assistance. When a late-stage hoarder is forced to clean up, it's often the county that's paying the bill. Social workers, building inspectors, and animal protection services are all paid for with tax dollars, so even people who aren't directly affected by hoarding are increasingly paying the price for it.

And last but not least, hoarders leave behind a legacy that causes a lifetime of pain. When a hoarder passes on and leaves a cluttered house, family members have to deal with it at a time when they are already raw and under tremendous stress, leaving the family unable to go through the natural phases of grief.

Too many families wait until the hoarding gets seriously out of hand before they start really pushing to fix the problem. Watching for the early warning signs is critical, and understanding the types and stages of hoarding outlined in Chapter 1 will make everyone's job much easier. Addressing hoarding sooner rather than later has tremendous short- and long-term benefits, potentially breaking the cycle of hoarding that causes so much grief. Since many of the mental situations associated with hoarding are serious and could be life-threatening, I advise my clients to consult with a therapist. This is important not only to deal with hoarding, but to improve the hoarder's quality of life in other related or unrelated areas.

When Not to Clean

SOMETIMES AN ASSESSMENT points toward not cleaning at all. If there is no pressure to clean coming from outside sources, like building inspectors or social workers, and the hoarder doesn't want to change, then it's often not worth the battle. Cleaning is a huge upheaval, and part of the assessment should be to decide whether or not it's worth it.

For example, Mario's daughter called me about her father's expanding car collection. Mario had been collecting antique, vintage, and junked cars for decades. He had easily a hundred old El Caminos, Thunderbirds, and other, mostly American models. The cars were piling up in the yard, and parts and paperwork were cluttering up the house where Mario lived with his wife.

Mario was eighty years old, and that car collection was his life's work. He was an old-school, macho "king of the castle" type guy, who was focused on being in control of his world. For Mario, his self-worth was deeply connected with his collection. Even after his daughter and wife talked to him about it, Mario had absolutely no desire to change.

The house itself was cluttered, but it didn't present any immediate danger. The piles were low, so they weren't threatening to topple over on anybody. The pathways were wide enough for emergency services to get in if they needed to, and all of the rooms were accessible. The major systems in the house worked—plumbing, heating, and cooling. Despite the clutter, the neighbors hadn't complained, and the county wasn't targeting Mario for a cleanup. There were no children in the house, and although

Mario's wife was frustrated by the mess, she felt that a cleanup would be too stressful for her husband.

After meeting with Mario and his family, I advised them not to clean up. A hoarder cleanup is exhausting for even a healthy, younger hoarder. A family could push its relationships to the limit, rely heavily on favors from friends, and likely spend a lot of money on a cleanup and therapy. In Mario's case, the stress would have been too much, going through his cars one by one, and the clutter in his house piece by piece.

With no outside pressure to clean, family members decided they would rather have Mario alive and hoarding than risk that the stress of the cleanup would do him in. They decided to let him live out his days with his collection, and plan instead for cleaning up after he was gone. I encouraged Mario's wife and daughter to continue to put gentle pressure on him to keep the shared space in the house clutter-free. But at eighty years old, Mario wasn't likely to change his ways. His wife, who loved Mario very much, decided to accept that he wasn't willing to change that one thing about himself.

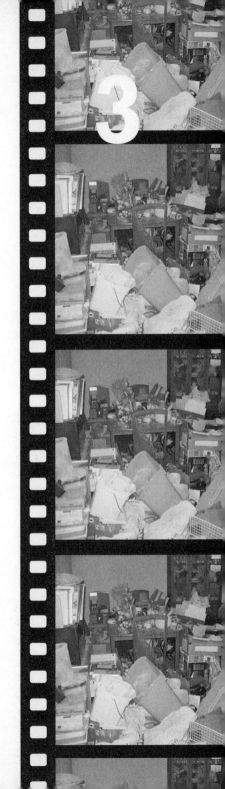

WHERE TO BEGIN

THE COLLABORATION:
A STORY WITH A SOMEWHAT HAPPY ENDING

Roger's two sisters were extremely patient while they figured out how to handle his hoarding issues. They spent more than two years assessing Roger's condition and exploring how to help him. During that time they went through what most hoarders' families experience. They were frustrated, confused, angry, and sad. They felt alone and ashamed. Despite that, they managed to stay positive during the process and focus on what was best for him.

Roger had been living at home in rural Georgia with his aging parents. With short-cropped hair and a full uncut beard that showed evidence of what he'd eaten on any given day, the forty-four-year-old was a tall, thin man with few social skills or contacts but an obsession for documenting his life—what he ate, where he went, what he wore—with the camera that he carried with him always. He even photocopied every single dollar bill before he spent it, notating the serial numbers and what he purchased. After his parents died, he withdrew from society even further, talking only to his family, mainly his older sister, Kathy.

Roger and his two sisters inherited the house and property. They all agreed that Roger would stay in the house until they could get it cleaned up and ready to sell and also find a new place for Roger. However, Roger was an extreme hoarder. While he had always hoarded in his room, when his parents died, within three years his stuff had spread into the rest of the large house, and he had also stopped taking out the trash.

At first, Kathy figured Roger was reacting to his grief. And she was right—Roger had been very close to his father, and that death sent him deep into mourning. Therapy was difficult to line up because Roger lived in a rural area, two hours from the nearest counseling services. His sisters gave him time and patience, figuring he would eventually stabilize on his own. They didn't push him, but they did keep saying, "Roger, you know we have to get this house clean."

The rest of the family was understandably frustrated when Roger couldn't seem to de-clutter the house, and in fact made it worse. But they kept talking to him, gently and with love, and finally they all agreed that they would pack up everything and move it out to the garage. Roger even helped. His sisters and their husbands spent four or five weekends filling up plastic bags and bins and moving them out to the garage for Roger to sort through later.

When the job was finished, Roger's sisters and their husbands went back home, a few hours away in the city. Roger was supposed to spend the next few weeks sorting through the items in the garage. Instead, in an unexpected change of heart, he started moving stuff back into the house. Another quick intervention followed, but left again on his own, Roger reverted to his old habits—bringing bags of things into the main part of the house and adding more to the clutter.

His sisters could have freaked out and verbally attacked Roger, understandably. They worked hard on two nasty cleanup jobs, and Roger had even agreed to both of them.

Everyone in that family was still reeling from the parents' deaths. They were all raw and could easily have been drawn into some emotional nastiness.

Instead, his sisters focused on trying to understand what was happening with Roger. They stayed patient and maintained loving spirits for a full two years after their parents' passing. They instinctively knew that something was wrong with Roger and that it wasn't his fault. They talked with friends, professional organizers, and cleanup people, searching for insight into the situation. They got some good advice on the logistics of sorting and organizing Roger's stuff, but not much help on his mental state.

After the second cleanup attempt failed, Kathy confided in her minister, and he put her in touch with me. She was so relieved to finally find someone who understood what the family had been going through, and to learn that they weren't alone. She thought Roger's problem was just that he was stuck in extreme grief. She had read a little bit about hoarding but hadn't talked with anyone who had firsthand experience.

Both of Roger's sisters realized that even as they were focused on supporting him, it was okay to talk honestly with him about the issue and their desire to help. They even told him that they were confused and frustrated when he moved his things back into the house from the garage. But they knew instinctively that pushing hard wouldn't work. It was more effective to understand him, and then do research and put together a plan for his particular situation.

The final chapter of Roger's story has not yet been written, but the progress that he and his family have made to achieve the best life possible for him is a testament to the patient effort of everyone involved—the immediate family, the professional cleanup crew, the family's pastor, and, of course, Roger.

WHAT WORKS, WHAT DOESN'T

The path to a successful cleanup is filled with obstacles. Just like a hoarder's home, finding the best way in and through the problem can be challenging. And the best intentions can often go awry.

A course like the one that Roger's family undertook can be a success story because it progressed, albeit slowly, as a collaborative effort. But far too many other well-intentioned and caring families don't fare so well, and the approaches they take to the problem are often misguided.

▶ The Ultimatum

"If you love me, you'll clean up the basement/attic/house."

"I'm leaving if you don't clear out this mess!"

Frustrated family members frequently threaten to stop communicating with the hoarder or, worse, cut all ties. They threaten to stop bringing the grandkids over to visit, or refuse to help pay the hoarder's bills.

Sometimes it seems like hoarders are choosing their possessions over the people they love most, which is why families are driven to these ultimatums. They want the hoarder to choose, but the hoarder can't—and they end up alone amid their junk.

Ultimatums arise from sincere and rational thinking. When Katrina's daughter threatened to keep the grandchildren from visiting, in the hope that she would see reason and put her house in order, what the daughter didn't comprehend was that Katrina wasn't thinking along rational lines. The ultimatum only created a goal in Katrina's mind that she could not achieve on her own. In her heart of hearts Katrina wanted to have a clean home and interaction with her grandchildren, but her brain couldn't process the idea of a cleanup like a normal person. She couldn't visualize the steps it would take to make this happen.

Once an ultimatum is thrown down, the hoarder who has been living in clutter and filth for years isn't going to be moved, but the person presenting the ultimatum now has to follow through. The truth is that few people want to cut off their family member—no matter how bad the circumstances. If Katrina's daughter did follow through and no longer brought the children to visit, she would only be breaking an important connection to someone she and her children love. Everyone loses.

Hoarders truly believe that they can clean up and will someday. When they can't, and when the people they love abandon them, depression kicks in. And then they start to wonder, why bother cleaning up? In their isolation, if they think that nobody cares, they can descend quickly into an ever-tightening spiral of depression and an expanding circle of mess.

However, for families who fall into the ultimatum trap, it's never too late to turn it around. A simple apology can work wonders. Even if a daughter doesn't really understand her mother's illness, she can admit that it's not laziness or obstinacy on her mother's part, show patience, and accept her, mess and all. All the while, she can be keeping in mind the story of Roger and his sisters, whose patience and careful planning eventually saw things to a positive outcome. Katrina's daughter has the opportunity to show her mother that she respects her intelligence and independence by allowing her to visit her grandchildren at their home. While the visit is on the daughter's terms, the cleanup will be on Katrina's because she understands that her family wants her to have a better life and that, together, they will find a way to achieve that goal.

Many hoarders have significant emotional and psychological issues, but they are neither stupid nor ignorant. In fact, most hoarders are very intelligent and can see through any mental games someone tries to play. Late-stage hoarders have already played those games on themselves for years. Forget the tricks. Respect the hoarder and spell out the game plan from the beginning. Straightforward conversations and respectful dialogue may start off slowly, but they can save years of wasted effort.

▶ The Secret Cleanup

My own family is a textbook case of how *not* to help a hoarder. When I was a teenager, I had a great-aunt who was a hoarder, although we didn't know that word at the time. She saved everything: newspapers, plastic bags, and paper towel tubes, to name some of what I recall seeing in her house. I am sure that she had every intention of recycling or donating stuff, but she just never got around to doing it. Every few years I would help her "clean up," which meant moving piles around and straightening them, because she didn't want to get rid of anything.

As the condition of my great-aunt's house deteriorated, her habits grew more bizarre—to the point where she was leaving the door open and peanuts scattered about for neighborhood squirrels to come in and eat. The family's concerns finally came to a head, and a secret cleanup was inevitable.

I can't even remember how the family got her out of the house overnight, but while my great-aunt was gone, my mom, aunts, and cousins descended on the house with a vengeance.

What my mother and cousins did made sense to all of us at the time. The cleaning process was similar to what I do with my clients today—sort through and organize everything, save the valuables, throw away the trash, and clean the whole place thoroughly. But the difference is that my great-aunt wasn't ready for anyone to go into that house. She wasn't part of that process at all. My family kept what *we* thought was valuable, not what *my aunt* thought was valuable.

Now, clearly her paper towel tube collection or the five thousand plastic newspaper bags probably belonged in the trash. But to my great-aunt, those were important items. She had spent at least ten years saving the cardboard rolls for the children's craft projects at church, and the plastic bags for the paper boy to reuse. She probably would have been okay with those things leaving the house if someone had agreed to take them where she intended. But the fact is that she came home and they were just gone, along with a lot of other things she was saving to use or donate. That was a big blow. Like my great-aunt, most hoarders have good intentions to give items they are saving to someone. It's in the follow-through that they drop the ball.

Unfortunately, a few of my great-aunt's possessions with sentimental value also went missing. She claims that they were thrown away, but we don't know if they were ever in the home in the first place. The items may have been stuffed deep inside an old purse, book, or plastic bag somewhere that nobody thought to open. I've learned that in working with hoarders, perception is reality. It doesn't matter if my aunt's items were in the house or not. What is important is that she thought they were and was devastated to not be able to find them.

Although my great-aunt's cleanup was more than fifteen years ago, I know that she hasn't forgotten what we did, because she still talks about the day that "those women" threw all of her stuff away. I hear from a lot of families who have gone in like mine did—brooms at arms and spray cleaners blasting. Or they threaten the hoarder with some terrible consequence if the house doesn't get clean. The stress on the hoarder in these situations is awful. This kind of intervention almost never works out and inevitably leaves families searching for help long after the hoarder has stopped talking to them and cluttered up the house again.

► The Ambush

The ambush is like the secret cleanup, except it takes place when the hoarder is around. And like the secret cleanup, it rarely turns out well in the long run. The fatal flaw of the ambush is that it pushes the hoarder to clean up before he or she is ready, and continues even if the hoarder wants to stop. In this kind of cleanup, the hoarder's defenses are as high as the piles of stuff in the house. Family members are insisting that the hoarder give up the one thing that that person depends on to feel safe. It's a lot to ask, and it's only going to work if the hoarder agrees that this behavior is causing serious problems. Usually, the hoarder does not think there is a problem.

Marcie, the shopaholic with the abusive husband, didn't want to let a cleaning crew into her house. Her son, Jordan, had called me about doing this job, and against my better judgment we arrived on Marcie's doorstop without first talking with her. (This was early in my cleanup career, and I hadn't learned yet that this type of cleanup rarely works.) Jordan said that he had not been in the house in almost twenty years. But he knew there was a big problem because one of his sisters had been allowed far enough into the foyer to see the extreme clutter on the main floor.

So I ended up waiting on Marcie's doorstep for two days. The first day I mostly stood on the porch and talked with her through a crack in the door. The second day we sat outside and visited for about an hour, and eventually Marcie opened the door so I could have a peek inside. It was an aggressive situation. What I could see were piles of clothes, trash, books, and stacks of shopping bags nearly to the ceiling.

Once we finally got inside, I judged that in terms of volume, Marcie's may still be in the top five most packed houses I've ever seen. I estimated that there were more than fifty tons of stuff, all piled up with little valleys that were used as walkways through each room.

A hoarder who is surprised by a crew of cleaners—be they family members or professionals—isn't going to react well. Even though Marcie eventually let us in, the two days I sat idle on the doorstep cost Jordan a lot, in more ways than one.

In an already unpredictable situation, if a cleanup crew moves too quickly, the hoarder's anxiety level rises. Because she was caught unaware, Marcie didn't really fully grasp what was going to happen. The three days that we spent easing Marcie into the idea of a cleanup were necessary, and even though she relented—and was even positive and upbeat for the most part—a confrontation with her husband brought the whole process to a halt.

Even under the best circumstances and with full support, a hoarder who isn't really ready may feel overwhelmed by the loss of control and just shut down. The more the hoarder feels threatened, the more likely it is that he or she will blow up and order everyone out of the house, and out of the hoarder's life. An ambush, in the end, simply confirms a hoarder's belief that people can't be trusted.

So, before any successful cleaning starts, the hoarder has to be ready. Family members are anxious to get started long before the hoarder is, but pushing just doesn't work. The best thing everyone can do is what Roger's sisters did: wait until the hoarder is ready, even if that takes years.

The waiting is critical, but it can feel unbearable. The anxiety and worry can pull families apart as they descend into bickering, blaming, and name-calling. Many stop speaking to one another. Ironically, all of that energy comes from concern—family members want to help, but without a clear plan, they get frustrated, and that frustration can come out in negative ways.

Fortunately, there is something more productive to do

during the waiting period. That's the perfect time to fully assess the situation, learning more about what causes it and what will be involved in a cleanup. This is a critical step toward building a cleanup effort that will stick. Hoarding cleanup is a huge job, so big that the people involved (including the hoarder) only want to do it once in a lifetime.

▶ The Intervention

The difference between an ambush or secret cleanup and an intervention is subtle but important. In an ambush the hoarder may be taken by surprise—or surprised when he or she returns home to see the deed has been done—but the hoarder does become part of the process. Interventions are usually forced when a state of imminent danger exists, or they are prompted by outside authorities. Whatever action is taken is done even though the hoarder may resist.

Some hoarding situations have strained a family's patience and resources to the breaking point—and an intervention is the only solution. The hoarder may have medical issues that mean he or she needs live-in or home health care. Or the hoarding progresses so far that local authorities—child, adult, or animal protective services—get involved. Under the worst circumstances, a building is condemned and the hoarder is forcibly removed. When a situation attracts that kind of outside involvement, it almost always involves a Stage 5 hoarder, who inevitably opposes a cleanup.

Given such extreme circumstances, the priorities set by family, friends, professionals, and the authorities move from simply supporting the hoarder to remedying a sometimes life-threatening situation. If the hoarder is facing the threat of having his or her children removed, then an intervention can be an option for putting the children first and finding a way to keep the family together. Usually there isn't any pretense that the hoarder is in charge of the process.

An intervention is the option of last resort and is usually a major decision. It can't be undone. Interventions should only be undertaken after serious thought and preceded by family meetings, consultation with a therapist or hoarding specialist, and discussions with the authorities. Aside from the physical issues of the cleanup, any concerns about the hoarder's mental state (depression, severe anxiety, or suicide) should be discussed with a therapist or specialist *before* the intervention. This is a really big deal, and an apology will not fix this decision after the fact. Families choosing this option need to appreciate and prepare for all of the consequences, including a complete rejection by the hoarder.

THE PLAN:
LAYING THE
GROUND-
WORK

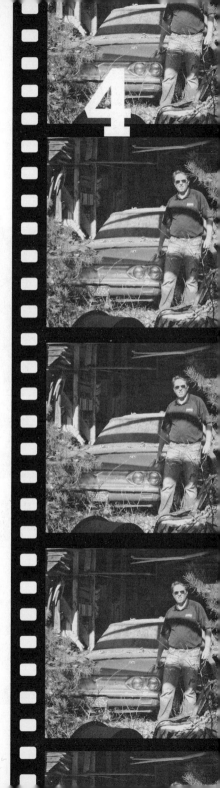

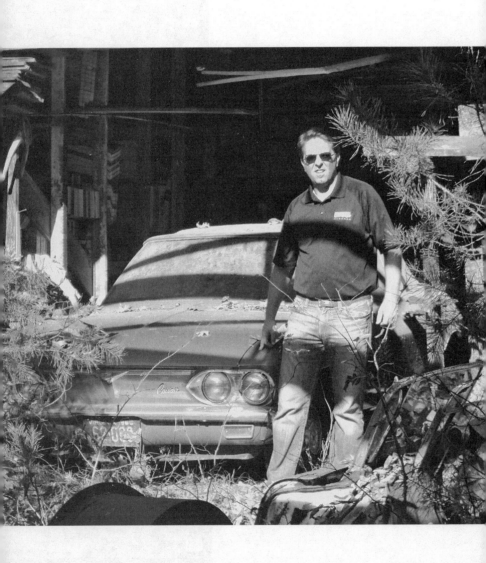

A cleanup is not a linear process, with one step leading neatly to the next. Every situation has its own course that requires a lot of patience, insight, and flexibility to navigate. But each cleanup needs to include some key elements in order to succeed.

Whoever instigates the cleanup, which in most cases is a close family member but which can be a friend or professional, will need to answer these questions, among others:

What am I dealing with in this situation?
Who are all the people involved? (Spouse, children, friends, and neighbors)
How can I get the hoarder on board with this cleanup?
Who will help me?
What are the expectations and goals we should have?
Is there a timeline that we need to follow for the cleanup?
What happens if the best-laid plans go awry?

ASSESSING THE CLEANUP

In the previous chapters of this book, we looked at the what, who, and why of hoarding, which provide the foundation for building an effective effort. Each situation is unique, but by identifying each part of the problem, you can determine the best overall approach.

The optimal cleanup looks like Roger's: The hoarder is involved because the family has patiently coaxed him in that direction. By the time he is ready to start, the family has a plan in place to be able to move ahead. Roger's sisters spent quality time assessing the situation and determining how the cleanup could take place.

Kathy knew what her parents' house looked like, but even she was surprised when the team showed up for the first cleaning. Roger's hoarding had spread throughout the house, and she wasn't expecting to see the extent of the clutter. Hoarding can move quickly after trauma.

Kathy knew that she could handle seeing her parents' house a mess. But some other family members might have gotten too upset, so it was important to make sure that everyone involved was prepared—and that whatever they might feel about Roger's part in creating the mess would be held back. If there is a family member who tends to get anxious or angry, is easily grossed out or overtly critical, that person is not the right one to assess the condition of the house or to help during the cleanup.

Someone does need to visit and determine the severity of the hoarding and what's being hoarded, so that the planner can figure out how other team members might be helpful. It's great if this is someone who can stay in touch with the hoarder and visit again, to reassess when cleaning time is near.

Even if Roger had not been cooperative, the plan that his family put in place was flexible enough—and they were patient enough—to let things take their course without undue pressure.

An important part of the plan—and perhaps the most obvious one—was how to actually accomplish the cleanup. Roger's family felt that they could take care of things themselves since many people were willing to pitch in to help. They had determined in advance what needed to be done. They knew the extent of the hoarding, what was being hoarded, and the potential value (or otherwise) of the stuff that filled the house. But, like all best-laid plans, when things didn't go quite as intended, they were able to step back, adapt their schedule, and give Roger the time and space he needed. As Roger's sisters learned, cleanup plans can sometimes take years to implement. Patience and acceptance are critical tools for anyone who works with a hoarder.

WHO'S AFFECTED BY HOARDING?

There is rarely an instance of hoarding that doesn't involve many people, directly or indirectly. The impact can be very far reaching, from family and friends to neighbors and even total strangers. Whoever initiates a cleanup needs to be aware of who falls within the circle of damage and how they are affected. As the attempts to organize a cleanup move forward, there can be many unexpected—and often unpleasant—surprises for the unprepared. On the other hand, knowing who is involved, even tangentially, in the hoarder's life can prove invaluable in formulating a plan that works to the benefit of everyone.

▶ Living with a Hoarder

The stakes are obviously high for people living with a hoarder. It's difficult—and futile—to give an ultimatum, such as "If you don't clean up, I'm leaving!" because someone who lives with a hoarder may have no other place to go. It's also personally risky calling the authorities, because they might threaten to take away the home. But at the same time it's impossible to escape the clutter.

People who share a house with a hoarder live in a perpetual state of struggle: On one side is their love for the hoarder and their need to have a home. On the other is the awareness that this isn't a healthy, or even safe, way to live. There are no easy answers to how to navigate this issue.

▶ The Hoarder Spouse

Nika, the clothes hoarder, had a husband who was furious about her hoarding. She not only bought clothes for herself, but for him as well—to show that she cared. But all Andre wanted was a clean house and more quality time with his wife. He didn't understand why she couldn't just get her priorities straight: If she really loved him, she'd try to get her hoarding under control. Because Nika seemed to be choosing her clutter over Andre, he felt alienated. He also felt trapped by the piles of stuff in the house, which was so cluttered that they couldn't even eat a meal together. The only space in the entire house large enough for the two of them to sit was on the bed.

Anyone who is married to a hoarder will benefit from therapy, since this situation goes far beyond just living in a messy house. Not only will therapy help in coping with a very difficult living situation, but it sets an example that can encourage the hoarder to seek treatment also.

At some point, the living conditions may just become intolerable. Then things really shift toward intervention, which is the action of last resort, because that's when the hoarder's spouse has to put himself or herself first. To maintain mental health and physical safety—and when all other courses have failed—the spouse may finally have to call the local zoning board or adult protective services. That's the time to be absolutely open with the hoarder and declare that the situation has become impossible and that a change is inevitable. It's not an empty ultimatum if the hoarder's spouse plans to actually follow up.

Imagining the worst-case scenario is scary: Authorities may condemn a house and forcibly remove the family. That is, however, one of the ugly realities of hoarding left unchecked. Just as with many other mental illnesses, hoarding can break families apart.

But even this drastic action can be done with love—or rather, tough love. A mother of a child who is hooked on drugs realizes that at some point she has to stop bailing her child out. It's the same with hoarding. Without appropriate action, a situation can turn into one of codependency or enabling. And sometimes the best course is a split. But it is important for both the spouse and anyone who is trying to initiate a cleanup to remember that the spouse didn't break up the marriage; it was broken up by the hoarder's unwillingness to try to change.

▶ Children of Hoarders

Children who grow up in hoarder houses aren't necessarily hoarders themselves. Beth was seventeen and so overwhelmed by her mother's lifetime of hoarding that *she* finally called child social services herself to see what her options were. Beth was leaving for college the following year, but her sister and brother were only twelve and ten. Beth felt obligated to save her siblings and hadn't been successful in her previous attempts to remedy the situation.

Child Protective Services advised that under such extreme circumstances the minor children could be removed, but they could not promise that Beth's siblings would be kept together, so Beth confronted her parents one last time with the threat of bringing in CPS. Her parents told her they would never speak to her again if she broke up the family, and Beth backed down.

Over the next six months nothing changed, and Beth canceled her plans to go away to school and enrolled at a local community college so that she could live at home and protect her brother and sister. But a few months after starting her freshman year, Beth dropped out of classes, started to drink heavily, and suffered from depression.

This story didn't have to have a sad ending. Children living with hoarders can't be expected to understand the nature of such an illness. And they shouldn't have to take on the responsibility for trying to remedy the situation, like Beth. Children like Beth feel ashamed, helpless, and marginalized. They grow up not learning how to clean or even tidy up. They never learn how to sort their possessions so that each goes into its own special place. They also don't learn how to set limits on the items they keep, and this lack of boundary setting can have ramifications throughout every aspect of their lives.

For anyone who takes on the task of spearheading the cleanup attempt, understanding the confusion and concern that children of hoarders have is an important aspect in formulating a plan that will have the best results and keep the family intact.

▶ Hoarders' Neighbors

No one wants to be the busybody neighbor. But in the case of Rick, the information hoarding professor, it took a complaint by a neighbor to the city officials to get him into the system and to get him help.

Social services are there to help people, not to punish them. Sure, other government bodies may fine a hoarder or take more drastic measures. But without that initial call, Rick's situation might have gone on for much longer, and with much more serious consequences. Even then, it was almost a year from that first phone call until the cleaning crew arrived at Rick's house.

Rick's neighbor didn't call the city constantly, and he didn't start a war with Rick. Rick was a nice guy; he probably wouldn't have lashed out, but some hoarders take great pride in antagonizing their annoyed neighbors. Sometimes that's the only power, and interaction with others, that a hoarder has. I have worked with hoarders who knew the local ordinances and laws better than the authorities did, and they delighted in pushing the limits.

Those who live near hoarders are stuck with smells, eyesores, and declining property value. Selling a home near a hoarder is doubly challenging. Unfortunately, there aren't many options in this situation. Knowing that the hoarder has a mental disorder doesn't really help minimize the problem.

A neighbor is rarely the person to spearhead an intervention, and legally speaking it's better to avoid any negative communications with a hoarder. The best approach is to contact city or county officials. And be aware that solutions won't happen quickly or smoothly, especially if the hoarding is advanced enough for neighbors to notice.

But for those who are tackling the issue, being aware of the history of interaction with neighbors—and, for that matter, with city or county officials—is essential. (We'll talk more about intervention by the authorities later on.)

GOALS AND EXPECTATIONS

Setting mutually agreed upon goals and managing expectations helped keep Roger and his family on track. (We'll talk more about setting goals collaboratively with a hoarder in the "Talking with Hoarders" section that follows.) Roger's sisters started off with the hope that he would end up in a clean house, living a normal life, pretty much as they did. But they quickly realized that Roger had such deep-seated issues that they had to adjust their expectations. Roger struggled in social interaction. At first we thought he might have Asperger's: His sisters said that while he had trouble making direct eye contact and carrying on a normal conversation, those symptoms had worsened after their parents had died. But as he bonded with our crew and his confidence grew, we realized that probably wasn't the case. Still, his sisters began to consider that Roger might never be able to recover completely from hoarding. Although he was a young man, his hoarding, and the deep-seated issues that had been driving it, meant that he might not be able to live completely alone and might never have a spotless house.

For a late-stage hoarder, "recovery" may only be a tidy room or two, with no more new items coming into the house. Such a hoarder may enjoy a safe, comfortable life but will probably never be completely clutter-free. Setting realistic expectations for both the helpers and for the hoarder is critical. In Roger's case it was important for everyone to adjust their expectations since the initial goal was to prepare the house for sale and move Roger to another home. His sisters stopped focusing on the ideal of Roger living alone, in a clean house, with a full-time job, even though Roger wanted to live alone and wanted to find meaningful work. They all came to accept that he could probably live alone with someone checking on him daily, and that he might find work through a program that included on-the-job training. They all agreed on achievable goals for Roger—not what most people would call "normal," but much better than the life he was living with his hoarding.

Jackson, the early-stage Blondie hoarder, along with his partner, Mike, had simple goals—to clean and repair Jackson's house, sell it, and help him learn some methods for limiting his hoarding. The overall goal was for the two to spend the rest of their lives together, and both were committed to doing whatever it took to make that happen. In this case, Jackson's outlook for recovery was very positive. He had strong support from Mike, and he had powerful motivation to change because he wanted the better future that was available to him.

Early-stage hoarders, like Jackson or Ellen and Brad, the couple we first met in Chapter 1, are more likely to achieve the goals of a clean house and a relatively normal life than more advanced hoarders. Hoarders like Roger and Margaret have either spent so much time in clutter or are carrying so much emotional or psychological baggage that it is usually not realistic to expect much more than a relatively safe environment in which they can live and enjoy some level of social improvement.

Success or failure will be defined by whether or not everyone meets those expectations, but even then a family's definition of success may change throughout the planning and cleaning process.

All goals (except in an intervention) should be about the hoarder. If a family's goal is to get that eyesore of a house clean so it doesn't embarrass them anymore, then clearly that's more about them and not about the hoarder. To get the hoarder on board, the goals need to be ones that that individual can buy into, like having a working kitchen, or being able to invite people into the house, or complying with health and safety standards that have been imposed by the authorities.

▶ Goals for the Cleanup

Jackson and Mike's primary goals focused on the elements of the cleaning. Together they wrote down their plan for who they'd hire to help, how long it would take to clean the house, how many days the team would work, and what days they would take off. They wrote down what Jackson would do with the clothing, collectibles, and other specific items that they'd decided to donate, sell, or toss.

Their plan even specified where the items coming out of

the house would be staged while Jackson made decisions about them, or while waiting for someone to take them to a donation site or sell them. Jackson's house didn't have much trash, but the plan addressed where things would go, who would haul them to the dump, and when.

Writing down these details was helpful because Jackson and Mike could refer to them during the cleanup in case there were misunderstandings. If Jackson suddenly decided to keep all of his Versace shirts, Mike could point to the list and say, "See, we agreed to sell those." They also shared the written plan with the cleanup crew before cleaning day so they could decide how to structure the job.

Sometimes a job is so big that it is like staging an event, and the logistics can be as overwhelming as the clutter itself. That's where a professional can help organize and carry out the cleanup.

▶ Goals for Health and Wellness

Wendy and Sam were an elderly couple who met late in life and started living together in Wendy's Stage 3 hoarded house. Wendy was a pill hoarder, and they both had multiple medical issues requiring pills, so the plan for them included health-related assistance. Since their medical concerns were being handled poorly, they needed a private duty nurse to help figure out what to do and how to schedule ongoing health care. Physically, they required clear access into and through all the rooms in the house, and they needed to have safety equipment installed, like grab bars in the bathtub. Of course, Wendy required some kind of counseling for her hoarding to ensure long-term relief.

Daisy, another aging hoarder, needed a plan that included counseling, advice about insurance, medical treatment, and medication. As with many elderly housebound people, Daisy, Wendy, and Sam potentially required home health care, and their places needed to be clean and safe enough to allow visits from medical aides and other helpers.

▶ Goals for Living

Kathy and Roger let the cleanup crew handle most of the logistics of their de-cluttering. In their plan they focused more on setting life goals: where Roger would live, what his life would look like, and how to get there. The goals were specific, like putting their parents' house on the market within four months, finding a new place for Roger to live by then, and having Roger apply for at least one job within a month after moving.

Deadlines are often essential to motivate people to get things done—whether it's the hoarder or the support group. But they should be reasonable. If a hoarder feels trapped by unrealistic timelines, he or she may shut down the whole process before it really gets started. (We'll discuss more about setting start dates in Chapter 6.) Even a Stage 5 hoarder house may take a professional crew only a few days to clean out, but this kind of short deadline increases a hoarder's stress level—and the risk that he or she will sabotage the whole enterprise. The hoarder isn't prepared to think in such a short time frame for such an emotional undertaking. Thirty to sixty days is easier to accept, and if the house gets clean faster, then everyone wins.

A late-stage hoarder in particular, who has been withdrawn from the world for years, isn't going to jump right back into the stream of society just because the house is clean. Life goals take time and patience to achieve. Advanced hoarders need help getting back into society, which may mean creating a structured setting in which they can learn to socialize again, such as volunteering their time and talents for a limited amount of time each week. Or encourage the hoarder to host a coffee at the house two months after the cleanup. The simple act of sending out the invitations reconnects the hoarder with lost friends, and commits the hoarder to following through with the event.

TALKING TO HOARDERS

The hoarder is a critical part of the goal-setting process, but those conversations can be tricky. Often a late-stage hoarder insists on living alone, but the family questions whether or not that's safe or even possible.

Sometimes, running the numbers can help make the decision. Look at what it will cost to fix up the house and make it safe. Often that's a huge amount. A family can put that in front of the hoarder, asking if the hoarder would rather spend money on that, or on a comfortable retirement home. The hoarder should make the decision. Usually there's not even a discussion because the cost to repair the home is more money than the hoarder has.

Both Roger's sister and Jackson's partner understood that in the beginning they had to set goals cautiously. Mike knew that Jackson's house could be clean in a few days, but he gave Jackson three months. Kathy set modest expectations for what Roger's life would look like after his cleanup. If a goal isn't achievable, then it becomes another failure for a hoarder (and the cleaning team and family). Instead, the cleanup needs to be their first success on the road to a new life.

Jackson, like most hoarders, didn't reach out for help himself. More often it's a concerned family member, friend, or social worker who calls a therapist or cleanup expert. When that happens, the hoarder generally isn't ready yet to start the process, and things play out with ultimatums, secret cleanups, ambushes, or interventions.

The best chance of creating a collaborative effort is to engage the hoarder early on. It's important that the right contact person (or people) talk to the hoarder. Since some kind of discussion may have already taken place, it's likely that the person closest to the hoarder has a sense of how open the hoarder is to talking about it. If those early conversations don't go well, then someone else might have to come into the picture.

It rarely works if a family member talks about how the hoarding affects others. Hoarders just tune out the chatter about how embarrassed others are, or how the hoarding affects property values. They already know that, but it's not enough to make them take steps to deal with it. Just as with fighting an addiction, the desire to change has to come from within.

▶ Starting the Conversation

In hundreds of hoarding jobs, I've never had one where a family member said, "Hey, I'm worried about you," and the hoarder responded, "You're right. Let's clean up!" There is always more than one conversation. The early ones may not go well, and the hoarder is probably going to respond with a lot of denial. It's important to just keep coming at it with the same message of love, concern, and offers to help.

Jackson told Mike about his "messy house" early in their relationship, but he never let Mike see it. They dated for about a year before Mike decided to begin pushing Jackson to open up about his issues. Although his hoarding was a big issue in his life, it didn't define who he was. Still, Mike's approach was the best. By confiding in Jackson that he cared about him and that he was concerned about the direction the clutter was going—and offering to help however he could—he acknowledged the problem but didn't force the issue prematurely.

Even with an early-stage hoarder like Jackson, it took a good six months of conversations for him to get comfortable talking about a possible cleanup. Mike would mention the house, and tell Jackson that they needed to deal with it to move forward. Jackson would agree in theory, but not set a date or timeline, and then Mike would back off. Or Mike would ask to see the house, but Jackson wouldn't commit. They were both nervous to press the issue because they didn't want it to interfere with their new relationship.

Mike kept working on Jackson. The two watched programs on television about hoarding, and they even came to hear me give a talk on hoarding at a home show in their town. Finally, Jackson agreed to talk to a professional cleaner. In the meantime, the two had moved into Mike's house, and they realized that they needed to sell Jackson's house.

Although Jackson had agreed to make the phone call, he kept putting it off. Finally, Mike encouraged Jackson to just pick up the phone and call. He reassured Jackson that he loved him and that he would be there to support him. Getting Jackson to make that call was the breakthrough that the couple needed. Once Jackson and I talked, Mike backed off and let us plan the cleanup.

In talking to a hoarder, it helps to focus the conversation on the clutter, not the person. Hoarders are then able to separate themselves from the mess. They can begin to think of themselves not just as a hoarder, but as a person who does (or can do) many other things as well. Most important, they can let go of the defensiveness that is preventing them from moving ahead.

This process can take months. Mike had an advantage in that he was living with Jackson and had time to build other aspects of their relationship. They spent a lot of fun time talking, cooking, and going out—activities that had nothing to do with hoarding. An important part of hoarding recovery is forming and growing outside relationships and finding healthy substitute behavior, which is what Mike and Jackson were working on without even realizing it. Then every once in a while Mike would mention the house. And when

Jackson tried to ignore it or change the subject, Mike would remind him gently that he was going to keep bringing it up until they dealt with it.

Kathy, Roger's sister, had quite different challenges. Of his two sisters, she had always gotten along with him best, so it was Kathy who was likely to get him to open up more in conversation.

After their parents' deaths, as Kathy and her sister were trying to deal with the estate, Kathy took the job of staying in touch with Roger, starting with weekly phone calls when she would always make a point to encourage Roger to take care of himself: eat well and get out of the house for some exercise or just to engage with other people at any level. She would also update him with any information she was getting on how to de-clutter and, of course, ask him when he thought he would be ready to start a cleanup.

Kathy knew her brother well and sensed that he would be comfortable at least talking about the cleanup with her. She had good instincts on how hard to push him and what he might be open to hearing. Most important, she cared deeply about him and was committed to his well-being over the long term. That's ideal for the contact person.

In conversations with hoarders, it helps to focus on the potential future, talking about how the hoarder's life might look later, or about the process of organizing and decluttering, which is much less threatening than using the term "hoarding." Talking about the future, but keeping the conversations positive and not about existing hoarding behaviors, is difficult but important.

Early-stage hoarders usually aren't in complete denial, so introducing the topic is not as difficult. With late-stage hoarders, one has to be more careful about language. Hoarders at this point don't trust many people, if anyone. They have been judged and rejected for hoarding more times than we can count. Their self-esteem is pretty low and they are emotionally fragile. Discussions with late-stage hoarders have to be carefully worded to be positive and supportive and avoid judgmental comments that will cause the hoarder to shut down.

While most initial contact is made by family members, sometimes an impartial outsider can talk about the hoarding with no emotions attached to those discussions. A social worker and a cleanup expert can be the bad cops to the family's good cops. The early involvement of a third party serves as a foil for the family members—someone for the hoarder to lash out at so the family relationships stay intact.

▶ When Is a Hoarder Ready?

Mike knew that Jackson was ready to call in help because Jackson had started talking about his future and about how he wanted his life to look. He confessed to Mike that he knew he had to deal with the house at some point. The two were making plans to share their lives together, and Jackson's house was a major obstacle.

Jackson was living in a "perfect past," with his Blondie memorabilia and a big collection of designer clothing. He was hanging on to a time that had made him happy, and he wasn't ready to let that go until he saw that he could have a fulfilling life in the present.

Hoarders are ready to tackle their issues when they start openly talking about what they miss out on in life, and what they want back. Instead of obsessing about why family members have kept them from seeing their grandchildren, for instance, they start to focus on the simple fact that they miss the grandchildren. They may admit that they want to see them, and at their own house instead of at the home of another family member. When the conversation changes from blaming others for the situation to expressing a wish for something positive, like more time with the family members, it's safe to give a little push—encouragement that says, "I am giving you my help, love, and support. If you really want to change, then now is the time." It can be as simple as asking, "What can we do to help you get your life back?" The hoarder has to decide what that action is.

▶ What Is a Hoarder's Role?

Candace, the former advertising executive we met in Chapter 2, was an exceptional worker who started her cleanup even before her helpers arrived. She talked with me on the phone, and because she was eager to start, we mapped out a plan before I visited the house. She had recently stopped drinking and said that she was ready to channel her energy into something positive.

Candace had boxes and piles of paperwork—mostly bills and other mail. She was willing to start there, sorting through each pile and box one piece of paper at a time, in search of old checks, overdue bills, and other important financial documents.

But Candace's OCD kicked in, and she wanted to make final decisions about every single piece of paper as she went through it all. In the interest of speed, it was a lot more efficient for her to group like items together, then sort through those after the major cleanup was over. So she put all of the bills in one bin, checks in another, family photos in a third, and trash in a fourth. By the time the cleaning crew arrived, three days later, Candace had already gone through ten boxes of paperwork completely on her own. She had four fifty-gallon trash bags of old mail to shred.

Brad and Ellen were also able to do a lot of the work on their own. I gave them a plan for staying clutter-free, which included a "ten-minute sweep" through the house every night. They focused on that and managed to get the house de-cluttered, and keep it that way.

Many hoarders can work hard all day long and keep working even after the cleaning crew has gone home. Others need supervision, frequent breaks, and take a more passive role in the actual cleanup process. In planning any cleanup it is very important to take into account both the hoarder's ability and his or her willingness to help. The hoarder should have a sense of being in control as much as possible, but that is determined by what he or she is physically and mentally able to do—and how sensitive the team is to the hoarder's needs, wants, and limitations.

How involved can hoarders be, and more important, how involved do they *want* to be? Can they carry boxes and items? Or should they sit quietly and "direct" the cleanup, deciding where things should go while others do the actual moving? Does the hoarder have health issues that may cut the workday short? When does the hoarder's day usually start—early or late? Empathetic team members will work with hoarders to build a plan that they feel good about.

I expect the hoarders I work with to give me 100 percent effort. Their 100 percent may not produce as much output as mine, but I want to know they are giving me everything they have. Sometimes a hoarder is so physically unwell or emotionally stressed or completely passive that he or she can only sit in a chair and say yes or no—and that's fine, as long as the hoarder is not showing signs of passive-aggression or simple resignation, which could result in some serious backsliding down the line.

In my experience, I have often found that hoarders who are argumentative or bossy—some might called it spirited— work hard once they've bought into the concept. But if a hoarder is particularly stressed or anxious, the cleanup may go more slowly, and the hoarder needs to stop frequently in order to get himself under control. This kind of development requires continuing patience and support.

► Sharing the Burden and the Rewards

During Roger's cleanup, his sister Kathy was always careful to say "we" when she was setting timeline goals and expectations. That way if the goals weren't met, she could say, "*We* failed," and share the responsibility with Roger. Hoarders have had so much failure in life already that they tend to easily assume more.

She was also quick to praise Roger, not the team, every time he took a step closer to the goals. Roger was certainly aware of his failures; he had been hearing about them his entire adult life. Kathy emphasized his accomplishments and abilities, and didn't dwell on his failings. She became his coach, and encouraged Roger to see himself as a strong person who had the power to change his life.

From the earliest planning stages, hoarders should feel like they are equals in the process, because that establishes mutual respect. It also confirms a shared responsibility for the whole process. Hoarders who feel equal to the cleanup crew know that there are expectations for them, and they are a lot more likely to meet them when treated with respect instead of contempt or sarcasm.

The cleanup person's job is to equalize the relationship through both words and actions. My crew shares stories of our own flaws and mistakes. When I tell stories about how my gambling got me into deep trouble, I follow that up by telling the hoarder that I know what it feels like to need help. I say that I'm there to offer support, not judgment.

We back that up with our actions. The house may be the hoarder's mess, but equality means that everyone—hoarder and crew—steps up and takes on the responsibility for the cleanup. It's one thing for cleaning helpers to *say* that they won't be judgmental, but it's much stronger to reinforce that by standing next to a hoarder and helping empty a refrigerator full of rotting food.

THE SECRET LIVES OF HOARDERS

Working side by side with a hoarder, without judgment, is like a continuation of the dialogue. It shows the hoarder that he or she has value and something worthwhile to offer to others.

▶ Control Is Critical

At the start of every job, my crew and I thank the client/hoarder for letting us help. This may sound odd, but we feel that it is important to acknowledge that the hoarder has made a choice to let strangers into his or her home, and that important decision initiates an entire change process.

For years hoarders have been told (or perceive that they have been told) that they are losers, slobs, messy, and out of control. They need to take control back in order to gain self-worth. Late-stage hoarders in particular have usually hit a point in life where they've failed at a lot of things. They've spent years beating themselves up. They've lost control of their house, of their possessions, of their relationships, and sometimes their jobs, diets, even personal hygiene. A cleanup is usually their first opportunity in years to impose control on their world, and to prove that they can be winners.

By having a sense of control over the cleanup, a hoarder earns back self-respect. Suddenly the hoarder has a team of supportive people in the house, listening to what the hoarder says. Instead of someone badgering the hoarder to throw items away, and complaining about the mess, people are handling things with care and asking where to put them.

Positive reinforcement throughout the process underscores the idea of the hoarder taking control. Hoarders aren't used to it, and it may take a while before they begin to hear and internalize compliments. But they need to feel confident, positive, and in control in order to maintain a clutter-free house.

THE PLAYERS: RECRUITING A TEAM

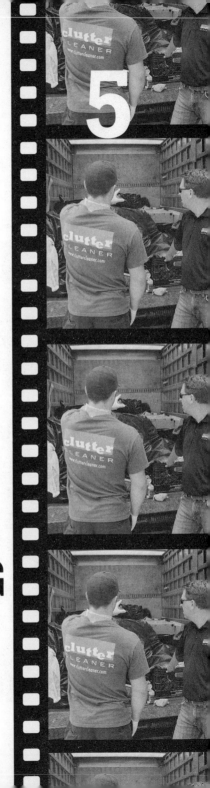

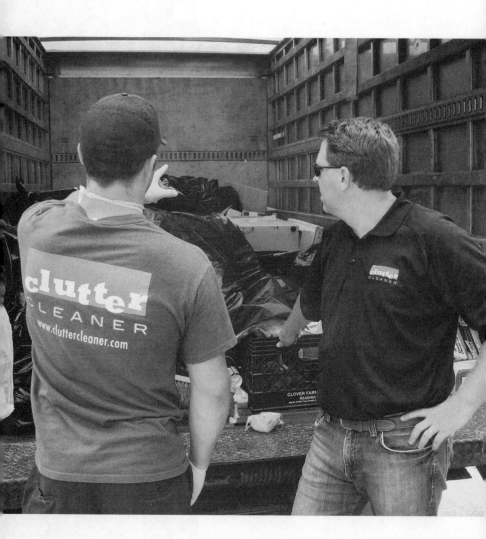

The best-laid plans for a cleanup are only as good as what can be achieved by the people involved. In the previous chapter, we touched on the importance of having the hoarder as fully engaged as possible and the value of a strong support group of family and friends. But many of the aspects of a hoarder cleanup are beyond the capabilities of this core group, which means experts and professionals will need to be engaged in order to deal effectively with the emotional, psychological, legal, and physical issues.

A CONCERNED—AND PERSISTENT—NEIGHBOR

Daisy was an eighty-five-year-old retired schoolteacher who had been living by herself on a fixed income for many years. As frugal as she was tiny, she had spent the last two decades hoarding everything and anything in her efforts to save money, and with the secret hope that some of what she saved might be valuable or useful someday. Someone once told her that she could turn her old newspapers in for cash, but the piles of paper had become unmanageable. She saved soda bottle tops to donate to fund-raisers. She "recycled" (reused) her adult diapers. Daisy was just trying to save every penny possible and, in the process, filled her town house to overflowing.

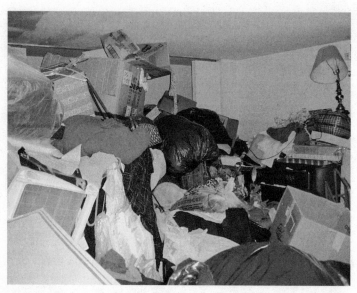

Piled almost to the ceiling, the cleanup crew was afraid of what they'd find under all of Daisy's clutter.

One morning Daisy's neighbor noticed the frail and elderly woman struggling with her front door, obviously trying to get back into her house. She asked if Daisy needed help, and kept asking what she could do even when Daisy insisted that nothing was wrong. Eventually Daisy admitted that she was blocked from reentering because something had fallen against the front door, and neither she nor her kindly neighbor was able to budge it.

When asked, Daisy told her neighbor that she had no family and really nobody else to call for help. But after a while, she said that perhaps her pastor would be the best person to contact. When her pastor arrived some time later, he could see, even through the front window, the terrible state of the house. He immediately made his first of many calls to Adult Protective Services to find out what help might be available. APS, in turn, got Daisy a social worker and put her up in a nearby hotel while they figured out what to do next.

The social worker became Daisy's main advocate. She put together Daisy's team, starting with county building inspectors. The inspection resulted in condemning the house, which, ironically, made Daisy eligible for county support services and triggered a local government process designed to fix up homes to allow residents to continue to live in them.

The social worker also connected Daisy with affordable medical care, so that she could get back on her medications and have regular checkups, both of which she had given up. Given her advanced years and late-stage hoarding, the social worker knew that Daisy wasn't likely to change her ways, so she didn't seek counseling help for her but rather focused on getting her a safe, clutter-free house, medical care, and a caretaker to help keep Daisy's life in order.

In addition, the social worker also engaged the services of a financial advisor whose job was to figure out Daisy's financial situation—how much money she had and what she owed—to see if she could continue to live on her own. And the social worker also called my company to clean out Daisy's house.

During the cleaning, the building inspectors checked in every other day to verify that the house was safe and to evaluate what repairs needed to be made. The financial planner came to collect important paperwork. The social worker stopped by each day to make sure Daisy was stable, emotionally and physically. She was also making sure that the cleanup crew was finding and passing along Daisy's family silver and lost checks. A rotating group of about thirty fellow church members came to work alongside my crew and help move boxes and haul trash. The pastor arranged for a volunteer construction team to repair damage from a two-year-old water leak. And the friendly neighbor who first discovered Daisy's problem popped in now and again to see how she was doing.

Daisy was one of the fortunate ones. Even though her

hoarding had gotten to such an extreme and she was having many other problems, she was lucky to have a watchful and helpful neighbor, a responsive pastor, and a superb social worker who were able to set the wheels in motion for a good outcome.

THE TEAM ROSTER

Every hoarding situation is unique. Who needs to be involved will depend on many factors. The most effective teams will include a range of participants, from family and friends, to social workers and community support services, to county officials and professional cleaning services. Depending on the circumstances, many of the services may be available at no charge or the cost will be underwritten by a government or social agency. Whatever the case, knowing who to call on and what you can expect from them can make all the difference in the success of any endeavor.

▶ The Family

Li was a widowed grandmother who was living alone in a crammed-full three-story house in rural Connecticut. She had always been a passionate shopper, but her hoarding had escalated after her children moved away and her husband died. Her eldest daughter, Sunny, along with her five sisters and brothers had spent years trying to get their mother to clean up. Nothing worked until the children figured out how to persuade their mother to act by presenting her with what amounted to a business plan—a plan that appealed to Li's innate sense of order, which had gone terribly awry. The plan identified the items they wanted to locate in the house, like some investment papers, family jewelry, and photographs. It pointed out how much more valuable the house would be if it was cleaned and maintained. And, after consultation with their mother, the children called me in.

The day my cleaning crew arrived, one of the sons took Li to his house to minimize her stress. Meanwhile, his wife and a sister stayed at Li's house, working alongside the cleanup crew, putting in twelve-hour days of sorting and hauling.

Although this was one of the fullest houses I've ever done—and chasing out a family of possums that had moved in was a bit unnerving—it was also one of the easiest. There was just no drama and no negativity from this family, which I've seen so many times. Families dealing with hoarding can dissolve into finger-pointing and blame under much less stressful conditions. Instead, Li's children were focused on what their mom wanted and needed.

Supportive, helpful family members are invaluable, as helpers and as emotional support for the hoarder. Family members who nag or blame shouldn't be part of the team. Hoarders have already had plenty of negativity; the cleanup should be as positive an experience as possible.

In Roger's case, his sisters decided that they and their husbands would be the core of the team. They undertook the research to determine who else could help: professional cleaners, therapists or social workers, and officials. They decided to include a Realtor to come assess the house and tell them what needed to be done before it could be listed for sale. After that they brought in some workers to estimate the cost of repairs.

Roger's sisters knew that helping their brother meant more than just getting the house cleaned. Sure, extra hands are useful on cleaning day, which is why they wanted a cleaning crew or other volunteers. But more important is the emotional work that continues long after the cleanup has ended. They knew that spending time with Roger afterward would be critical to helping him learn how to socialize again and encouraging him to find a more positive activity to replace his hoarding behavior.

Roger's sisters understood instinctively that if they started with Roger and then quit, it would become yet another loss and failure for him. They all committed to stay the course because to start and then abandon their brother would have been worse for him than to not start at all.

▶ Friends, Neighbors, and Coworkers

During Daisy's cleaning, she was visited by the neighbor who had helped her when she got shut out of the house. The neighbor had never seen the inside of Daisy's house and was shocked at how bad the hoarding was. Although the neighbor asked how she could help, Daisy didn't want her involved in the cleaning itself.

A cleanup is deeply personal for the hoarder. The best team members are close family members, and after that the circle can widen to include specialists who can help with certain aspects of the job. Inviting acquaintances, coworkers, or extended family to help usually adds to a hoarder's anxiety level. The hoarder is already worried about being judged by family and doesn't usually respond well to opening up this secret life to the world at large.

The members of the team should be as discreet as possible about the cleanup. There are likely many acquaintances who don't know about the extent of the hoarding, and it would be inappropriate for anyone involved to betray the hoarder's confidence and risk changing the nature of the hoarder's relationship with coworkers, neighbors, or others for the worse. There are always jobs that extended family or friends can do that may not directly involve the cleanup per se, like bringing meals, making phone calls, or running errands.

Once the cleanup is done, a hoarder will need relationships that are based on something besides hoarding. Having "outside" friends that draw a hoarder in healthy new directions is an important element of long-term success.

For a family trying to save money on a cleaning, a team of trusted volunteers can work, but they should be chosen carefully and with the consent of the hoarder. It's important to remember that this is the *hoarder's* team, not the family's team. The hoarder will be spending long days with this crew, making tough decisions on very personal items. The hoarder needs to feel safe and comfortable. By the end of the cleanup, these team members will essentially be this person's closest friends, and it is important that they stay in touch with the hoarder post-cleanup.

▶ Clergy

In Daisy's case, that pastor at the church that she had attended for more than a decade acted as an informal social worker early on. He had her best interests in mind, and he took the time to find out what support was available to help her. He was also the only person who had her immediate trust, and he was able to pass that to the others he brought into the cleanup. It's important to take advantage of "trust swapping" if the hoarder is already connected to someone, because establishing trust takes a long time.

Members of the clergy and other spiritual advisors are often trained to help with both emotional and logistical support. And because they are already trusted by the hoarder, they become important in the short term to help get things moving—and as ongoing support for the hoarder. A priest or minister has access to lots of local resources, not just city programs but also private programs or even individuals who want to help in some way. Many churches and other religious institutions have special support for those in need, like temporary housing quarters, feeding programs, or volunteer construction crews like the one that repaired Daisy's house.

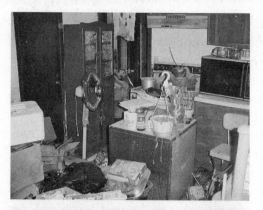

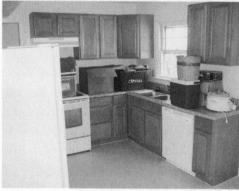

In addition to the professional cleanup crew, Daisy's kitchen required a lot of labor, much of which was provided by supporters from her church.

Daisy's pastor also spoke from the pulpit about her need, and recruited a revolving team of volunteers who helped with the actual cleaning.

A hoarder's place of worship can also help reconnect him or her to the community at large. Daisy, for instance, volunteered for the feeding program at her church. Working with people in need helped Daisy feel good about herself and realize that she was more than just a hoarder. She felt confident that she was working toward building a worthwhile life, where she could help people and connect with others.

Even hoarders and families who aren't strongly religious might consider reaching out to a priest or minister for help and information about community support. Getting involved in a church will also create a support network for when the cleanup is complete.

▶ The Therapist

Thalia is the Stage 5 hoarder from Pennsylvania who had been a political volunteer—and saved pretty much every bit of paper from every campaign on which she had worked. (She is also our case study for high anxiety in Chapter 2.) During her cleanup, she asked for frequent stops and retreated to a bedroom. Her family members told us that her behavior was pretty typical, that she had been under a therapist's care off and on for years, and that she had a history of suicide threats and attempts.

The second day, Thalia fell completely apart. As soon as the crew approached her to make decisions about her stuff, she panicked. She ran outside and locked herself into her car, which was also full of bags, clothing, and memorabilia. As we stood outside the car and tried to get her to open the door, she started trying to open a bottle of pills, threatening to swallow them.

Because of Thalia's unstable mental state, we made sure that her therapist was on call during the cleanup, and it was the therapist who was able to talk Thalia out of taking the pills, and out of the car. At the therapist's insistence, Thalia was committed and spent the next few days in the hospital.

As extreme as Thalia's case may be, it is not uncommon for advanced hoarders to be wrestling with some deep psychological issues that will surface during the stressful time of the cleanup. Any hoarder with a previously diagnosed or suspected mental disorder, like OCD or depression, should have the support of a good therapist whose professional training will make him or her a critical and still impartial member of the team. In many cases, the therapist not only helps the hoarder directly but can manage the high emotions of the whole team.

▶ The Social Worker

Sam and Wendy met at church when both were in their seventies. When they fell in love, their children didn't have a problem with their racial difference. What shocked Sam's family was the condition of Wendy's house. When Sam moved in, the house was so cluttered and decrepit that they worried about his safety.

Both Sam and Wendy were strong-willed people. Sam made a commitment to stick with Wendy even though she simply wasn't interested in undertaking a cleanup. In frustration, Sam's daughter finally called the county to report Wendy's house. While this move could have alienated Sam from his daughter, it turned out to be the best move because it brought an empathetic social worker into the picture.

The social worker determined that Wendy and Sam were capable of living independently, and since they were adamant about staying in the house, she took steps to help them with a cleanup.

The social worker was also instrumental in getting Wendy and Sam the medical attention that they both needed. Sorting out the prescription drugs was a major issue. From old aspirin to expired heavy-duty narcotics, Wendy had hoarded old medications, which she took on her own judgment whenever she felt ill. She also kept empty bottles so that she would have a record of her medication history. The social worker got a doctor to visit and explain that medicines lose their effectiveness after time, and that her doctors would all have her medication records on file, so she could throw away the old bottles.

During the cleanup, the social worker checked in every day or two to make sure that Sam and Wendy were holding up during the difficult process. If new problems had cropped up, she would have been the go-to person to coordinate additional resources and support.

With the help of the social worker, the cleanup crew was able to get Wendy and Sam's immediate cooperation. Social workers not only have the confidence and respect of their clients but give an air of urgency to the situation. And, trained as they are, they know the best and most effective ways to get help.

▶ Child and Adult Protective Services

Child and Adult Protective Services are social workers who specialize in aiding children or seniors who are living in hazardous conditions. They can rally the same level of resources and support as a general social worker, but are more focused on children or seniors in need. It's important to remember that these, or any, social workers are there for the person in need, which means they may not always do what family members think is best. They are focused on the *hoarder* or the people directly affected by the hoarding.

▶ City, County, or State Officials
The Building Inspector

Hoarders won't be the ones to call in a building inspector to condemn their own houses. But ironically, once city or county officials get involved, a battery of municipal programs kicks in to help the homeowner. The city or county doesn't want to own houses, they want to help homeowners fix them up and keep them.

Rick, the retired professor who hoarded paperwork, was living in a firetrap filled with twenty-five years' worth of papers, and the room he called his library had also been damaged by a years-old water leak. Rick's sister called the county because she was concerned about Rick's living conditions. The city inspectors condemned the house not only because it was a firetrap but also because they found high levels of black mold.

After blocking off the room with the hazardous mold, which would be handled by a special crew, the inspectors checked in every other day during the cleaning to make sure no new hazards were uncovered. In hoarder houses, the clutter covers up a multitude of sins, including structural damage that's not even visible until piles of stuff are removed from the house.

When a city or county official visits a house to evaluate the condition, the official writes a report with a list of things that have to be fixed and issues a warning. The homeowner is supposed to attend to those items on the list by the official's next visit, usually thirty days later.

Because die-hard hoarders don't usually comply—or do so halfheartedly—the next inspector invariably issues another warning. This may go on for some months, and if the homeowner makes any effort at all, then the inspector will postpone action, give the hoarder a provisional pass, and allow the homeowner to stay in the house, with the promise that the work will be done. For the house to actually be condemned, the inspector has to have made many visits over a long time period. But even once a house is officially condemned, things don't necessarily start moving quickly.

A property that has actually been condemned is on the building inspector's radar as long as that same homeowner is in the house, even once it's cleaned up. If the hoarder leaves something in the driveway, a neighbor's phone call will usually trigger a quick visit. Even without anyone filing reports, the inspectors will be visiting that house a few times a year just to make sure it's staying clean and habitable.

Pest or Animal Control

Michelle had a hoarding problem that had become so bad that Child Protective Services had removed her two middle school–aged children and city authorities had determined that the house had to be cleaned immediately. In every room of the house newspapers were stacked about seven feet high, making access throughout the place difficult. But the real problem was the mice that were living in the clutter. The pest control man said that with close to three thousand mice, it was the worst he had ever seen. Our cleaning crew eventually filled two fifty-gallon trash bags with dead mice.

Michelle had been living in those conditions for years, and like many hoarders she was not a healthy woman. She was rail-thin, with her clothes sagging off her narrow shoulders. She coughed a lot, and her skin was dull and flaky. I don't know if any of her health issues were caused by the mice, but it's not a healthy environment for anyone.

Vermin like mice, rats, and cockroaches are common in hoarder houses, and a house like Michelle's needs to be treated before cleaning can begin. These creatures carry viruses dangerous to humans, including hantavirus and Lyme disease. Some viruses are passed not by direct contact but just through rodent droppings and saliva. A mouse infestation like Michelle's also increases the risk of children developing asthma.

If there are a lot of pets in a house, animal control people may be a necessary part of the team to make sure the dogs, cats, birds, snakes, or other pets are taken to a shelter where they have food and space. There, they can be evaluated for health problems and given medical care. If the hoarder can't care for the pets after the cleanup, then animal control has the resources to find them good homes.

The Police

There are many circumstances before and during a cleanup that might involve the police. When we were working with Marcie, the shopaholic whose husband turned out to be abusive, things came to a head when the husband took a swing at me. It seems that he didn't take too kindly to his wife's realization that part of her hoarding problem may have stemmed from his abusive behavior. After that, we decided that if we were to return to the house, we'd need some police oversight. As it turned out, he beat us to the punch: Marcie's husband took out a restraining order preventing us from coming back to the house.

Don, on the other hand presented a very different sort of situation that required police intervention. An overweight, ex-military guy who had retired from his civilian job working in security, Don had suffered a heart attack but managed to call 911. After the emergency services crew picked him up and got him to the hospital, they called county officials about the house, which was in a terrible state. A few months later, county officials called in my cleaning crew. Almost immediately we found a loaded handgun underneath a pile of clothing. Don admitted that one wasn't the only weapon in the house, so we stopped cleaning and called the police. They discovered seventeen guns and thousands of rounds of live ammunition. We then continued our work, only to uncover more ammunition and weapons, and we had to periodically call the police back in to handle the situation.

Will's case was equally troubling. He was a hoarder recovering from surgery who needed his house cleaned out enough to allow home health care to get in and help him. We began cleaning and almost immediately started finding pornography. That's not unusual; we find all sorts of private things when we clean, and we are usually very discreet. Will was apparently obsessed with famous cartoon characters.

He had a vast collection of mermaid drawings and other characters, all in revealing and compromising positions.

The deeper we got into the house, the more disturbing the pornography became: child pornography and snapshots of Will with girls who looked underage. This went beyond "private" into illegal, and so we were compelled to call the police. Will ended up recovering from his surgery while serving a three-year prison sentence.

Police are valuable members of the team whenever there is violence, or the threat of violence. And they are mandatory when there is dangerous or illegal activity, including drugs, firearms, child pornography, or abuse.

▶ Professional Cleaners and Junk Removers

The worse the hoarding case, the less likely family members or friends can handle the cleanup themselves. Professional cleaning services can be involved to whatever extent necessary, from simply hauling away trash to cleaning the entire house and arranging for specialized support, including therapy. A reputable cleaning company trains its staff to handle everything from hazardous waste to valuables as well as to work appropriately with the hoarder or other helpers.

If a family feels that they can handle the work themselves, then they can still hire the cleaning service to create a plan and a list of necessary materials. Or they can work alongside the professionals. But if a house shows signs of a high level of hoarding, the unsafe conditions may require the intervention of professionals.

▶ Appraisers or Auctioneers

Jackson was unusual in that his Blondie collection and designer clothes actually had some value. He had autographed Blondie memorabilia and rare collectibles. Jackson and Mike didn't bring in an appraiser because a quick scan of eBay showed them that the collectibles were fetching pretty good prices and a call to a consignment shop determined the value of the clothing. But under other circumstances, a visit from an appraiser or auctioneer might be a good idea.

What I see is that 99 percent of the time the collection has little or no value. But hoarders are convinced that they are sitting on a gold mine. Bringing in an impartial third party can clear this up, because it's harder to argue with an expert. But the house has to be fairly clean before the appraiser is brought in or the appraiser may dismiss everything as "messy junk" without making the effort to really see what's what. Since most appraisers charge by the hour, it's cost-effective to have the "valuables" already pulled out and boxed up before the visit.

Because most collections are relatively worthless, be prepared for this additional emotional blow to the hoarder. It's best if an appraiser comes to visit the hoarder and maybe one other sympathetic family member. Families can be tempted to say "I told you so!" to a hoarder when the hoarder learns that that extensive angel figurine collection isn't worth any money. That can be a really hard moment for a hoarder who has a lot of money and emotion invested in the collection, and the hoarder needs someone who will understand and be kind and positive.

The auctioneer, on the other hand, may take a wide range of stuff—both valuable and not—and make arrangements to dispose of it in the most profitable way possible. The auctioneer will, more often than not, take a large batch—except real trash—and sell it off in job lots or individual pieces. It is worthwhile for auctioneers to get the most they can for everything since they are usually taking a percentage as their compensation.

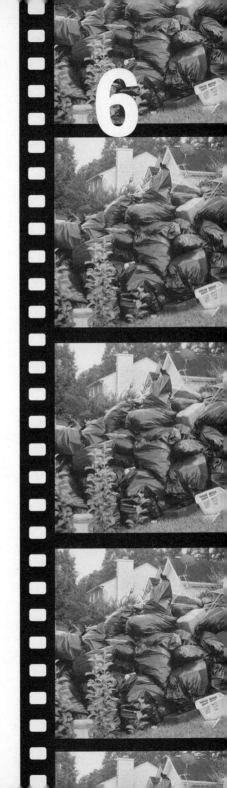

THE
CLEANUP

Aimee lived in a two-bedroom condo in New England. She had worked as a high-end fashion model when she was younger, but by age forty-eight it was impossible to see her fine bone structure or once-toned figure. Aimee looked like a stereotypical hoarder: overweight, with pasty skin and curly black hair streaked with gray. She spent her days in bed, drinking cans of nutrition shakes, giving herself insulin shots, and sliding to the edge of the mattress to go to the bathroom.

Until she started confining herself to the bed, Aimee had been a clothes hoarder whose obsession had gotten out of hand about eight years earlier. Aimee had kept the clothing from some of her modeling jobs, samples that the studios had given her as well as clothes that she had bought. She had about four hundred pairs of shoes and more than a thousand purses. Her collection was stacked in piles around narrow walkways through the house. On top of that was another foot of trash, from the point about two years earlier when Aimee gave up the hope of de-cluttering and just started tossing everything onto her piles.

The stink from the urine and feces had gotten so strong that neighbors had called the city to complain. Building inspectors visited and condemned the house, but they told Aimee she could keep it if she cleaned up and it passed reinspection within ninety days. The city hired us to work with Aimee.

No matter what the stage of hoarding, what the hoarder hoards, or what other mental disorders might be involved, hoarder cleanups all start with the plan. Cleanup day is when the rubber finally meets the road. The team meets outside the house to assign jobs, grab trash bags, and dig in. Each stage of hoarder has different issues, and any plan should be flexible enough to take that into account.

From my point of view, the actual cleaning may be the easiest part of this process. For a team that has done its research and put together a good group with a workable plan, cleaning will go surprisingly smoothly. It's the mental and emotional preparation with the hoarder that's tough, along with the hand-holding and guidance during and after the process. The cleaning itself is just a matter of sorting items into piles to keep, donate, sell, recycle, and trash.

STAGE 1: BRAD AND ELLEN

Their hoarding was so early-stage that Brad and Ellen decided to try cleaning it themselves, without a professional organizer or a cleanup service. They called me for a consultation, and after walking through the house I wrote up a plan for them that focused on their main problems: Brad's computer stash; Ellen's teaching supplies; food; and the children's clothes and toys. Brad and Ellen set aside a weekend, sent their three young boys to Grandma's, and bought a few boxes of heavy-duty trash bags.

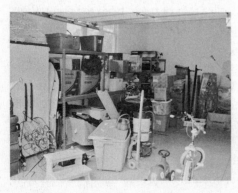

Brad and Ellen's garage before the cleanup. Simple Stage 1 that just needed some rules for organization.

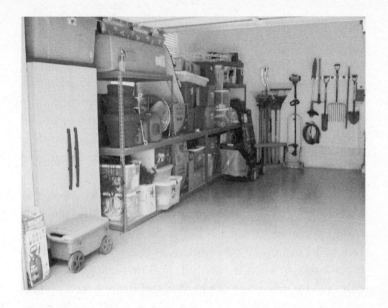

They finished the house in two days, following the plan guidelines. Brad started with his computers. He had saved them to fix up and donate, but he realized that he didn't have the time. Instead, he found a computer recycling company to collect them. Ellen went to work on her teaching supplies. Once she started sorting through the material, she realized that a lot of it was already out of date. Also, advances in technology meant that kids were working from computers, not construction paper. She filed away her teaching plans and some supplies, but she tossed her outdated workbooks. Getting rid of the old computers and Ellen's teaching materials cleared a lot of shelf space for toys and books in the kids' basement playroom. Part of this family's goal was to begin showing the kids, all under age six, a new skill: how to stay clutter-free. And Brad and Ellen's efforts were a major step toward that goal.

Ellen went through the boys' clothes and gave away anything worn, stained, or out of style. She boxed up the nice clothes that were too small and took them to a consignment shop. Brad loaded his extensive music collection onto his computer and then donated his huge stack of CDs. With the rooms emptying out, the couple started working on the odds and ends cluttering up the dresser tops, chairs, and corners. In the kitchen, Ellen and Brad were surprised by how much out-of-date food they had in the refrigerator and freezer, and they threw it all away. Cans and boxes older than six months but still good were donated to a food pantry.

Ellen continued to sort out clothing, books, toys, and knickknacks to bag and take to a donation site. She was training herself to not stack piles, but to place the donation items in a box by the front door that was small enough for her to lift when it was full. Follow-through is a difficult task for any stage of hoarder, so Ellen worked on taking that box to her car as soon as it was full so she could then go directly to her preferred donation site at the end of the day.

It took Brad and Ellen a day and a half to get the rooms completely de-cluttered. Then they were able to give the house a deep cleaning. They were shocked by the amount of dust and cobwebs that they had all been living with and breathing. Seeing how much underlying dirt had accumulated made them resolve all the more to stay de-cluttered.

Their cleanup plan also included follow-up rules to which Brad and Ellen could refer when they were cleaning, or making decisions about bringing in new things. For a Stage 1 hoarder the focus is less on the actual cleaning, which goes relatively quickly. The important thing is to learn and apply new skills. Early-stage hoarders have the same attachment to possessions that more advanced hoarders do. But because Brad and Ellen had fewer items, and hadn't been living with the behavior as long, it was easier for them to de-clutter, break bad habits, and learn better ones.

STAGE 2: JACKSON

Once a plan is in place, everyone has to agree to the start date. Jackson, the Blondie hoarder, tried to cancel his cleanup twice. The first time he said he was sick. The second time he admitted that it was nerves. We convinced him to let us come just to see the house for an assessment, and told him that he could change his mind about the cleanup at any time.

As the new start date approached, the team behind Jackson began to assemble the supplies and services that would be needed—and had other supporters on call, such as repair and renovation people, just in case. Most important, Jackson's partner, Mike, was preparing for Jackson's increasing level of anxiety by being patient and reassuring.

Because of the sheer volume of clutter in Jackson's house, and because he had been hoarding longer, he needed more workers and supplies than Brad and Ellen did. With his cleanup crew of three hired workers, Jackson had extra muscle for hauling away his bags of clothing and memorabilia. He also got one-on-one time with a professional cleaner to help direct him. Jackson was willing and able to learn new habits for decision-making and sorting, but he needed reminders and redirection during the cleaning. Basically, he needed a little coaching.

Jackson's house wasn't dirty, just cluttered. We started in the living room—the biggest room, and the easiest since it was filled with lots of empty cardboard boxes. In any cleanup, the house gets messier before it gets tidy, and the growing mess can be alarming to the hoarder. Finishing the first day with a large, clean room is very rewarding and motivates everyone to keep going.

Recycling the empty boxes opened up a large part of Jackson's living room and made space for staging items that needed to be sorted through. Then we moved on to making some easy decisions on donating items.

First, we worked on sorting everything in the house into piles of like items—clothing, collectibles, toiletries, bedding, kitchen equipment, and so forth. Jackson's plan was to then sort through each of those piles to make "trash," "keep," "donate," "sell," and "maybe" piles. Although the "maybe" pile grew, we knew he wouldn't keep all of those items. Jackson was beginning to understand what was important and what wasn't, and when he went back to the "maybe" pile, we were sure he would realize that some of these things weren't worth keeping.

The first morning, we discovered a box of Cher's doorknobs. Yes, Cher's doorknobs. Jackson had bought them online, when Cher was renovating her house. They were strange and beautiful—a dragon's paw, a crystal ball, and other assorted shapes and styles. Jackson agonized over whether or not to keep that box, and then started to panic about his entire house, realizing that he had seven rooms filled with similar items he had to make decisions about.

The doorknobs went into his "maybe" pile, along with several other things, and finally Jackson began to see that the cleaning process was manageable and that he was able to overcome his fears. When Mike showed up with lunch on the first day, Jackson realized that he had the support he needed, and that Mike wasn't going away. Jackson's anxiety went down to almost nothing, and he rolled on through the house.

During the sorting, we made a rule for Jackson that anything he decided to move out of the house had to leave *that day*. If he wanted to give a leather coat to a neighbor who had admired it, that was fine, but he had to contact the neighbor and get it to him right away. Otherwise, it went to the donation site at the end of the day. The "donate" and "trash" piles got hauled away daily so that Jackson wouldn't be tempted to pull items back out later that night. Mike listed the "sell" items on eBay within a day or two. Jackson saved the "maybe" items to sort at the end of the cleaning.

To keep on track, Jackson reminded himself repeatedly of the goal to sell his house and move in with Mike. Whenever he debated about an item, he asked himself if it fit his goal. The impressive Cher doorknobs were ultimately kept because Mike and Jackson agreed that they could go in their new place—and besides, they were real conversation pieces. But most of Jackson's clothing and other collectibles did not fit his goal—he had already moved enough clothes to Mike's house, and they only had room for so much Blondie.

Three days into the cleanup, Jackson had repeated his new sorting process so many times that it had become his new habit. Without any prompting he was making quick, confident, and accurate decisions about items—whether to keep, sell, donate, or throw away. Because he was so highly motivated, Jackson was able to work independently. We decided that he could finish the last two rooms by himself, and so my crew and I packed up and left Jackson and Mike with the confidence that this was a success story.

STAGE 3: RICK

Rick, the retired professor/information hoarder in the suburbs of Washington, DC, whose house was too far gone for him to even consider cleaning it alone, had an additional complication for the cleanup on top of the volume of paper. Physically, there were high levels of mold in the house, and mentally there were signs of dementia. The damage to his house was so extensive that Rick needed a large team that included building inspectors and construction workers, specialists to deal with the mold, a document disposal company with an industrial shredder, and a cleanup crew equipped with respirators and protective clothing. Rick's deeply ingrained hoarder habits and dementia indicated a slower and potentially more expensive cleaning.

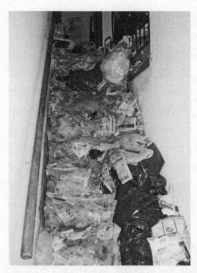

Layers of paper—old newspapers and junk mail—carpeted the stairs in Rick's Stage 3 home.

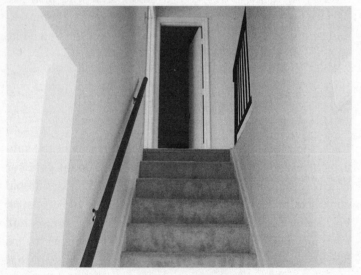

Rick's stairway after the cleanup.

Rick and his sister, who had actually instigated the cleanup, met my cleaning crew at 9:00 a.m. on the agreed-upon start date. Rick hadn't wanted the neighbors to know that a hoarding cleanup company was at his house, so we arrived in an unmarked truck after the neighbors had all left for work.

Rick's house was filled with old mail, files, and magazines. There was a two-foot-high paper "carpet" in the living room. In the kitchen, paperwork covered the countertops and flowed off onto the floor. The dishwasher didn't work, and the oven was filled with books and stock certificates. A mattress was propped up in the hallway, also covered with paperwork. The bedrooms weren't as full of paper, but clothing and trash littered the floors, and Rick's mattress smelled like it had been soiled.

The cleaning crew started in the living room, picking up papers a handful at a time, and sorting through them to put some in boxes to keep and the rest in heavy-duty trash bags to be dumped. They were looking for the items that Rick wanted to save, including the deed to his house, some retirement checks, and family photographs. He wanted those and his academic papers packed into boxes for him to sort through later.

Rick sat on a stool in the kitchen, picked through boxes of paperwork, and answered questions about what to do with other items the crew found as they worked their way deeper into the house, like the mattress (keep), a second microwave (donate), an exercise machine (donate), and dirty clothing (wash and donate). Just as I did with Jackson, I helped Rick when he got stuck on wanting to keep an old magazine or a piece of junk mail. I reminded him that he had decided that he wanted to sell his house and move in with his sister, and this was the path toward his goal.

After two hours, Rick was exhausted and overwhelmed. His sister took him out for coffee to give him a change of scenery. With Rick's permission, the crew kept working. While he was gone, we put aside anything that we felt would require a decision from him.

Rick, his sister, and the cleaning team worked through the house for three days, taking frequent breaks. The crew made ten trips to the county recycling station to dispose of twenty-four tons of paper. The building inspectors dropped by every other day, checking to make sure we hadn't uncovered more mold and that the floors and walls were in safe condition.

During the cleanup Rick was forgetful, often asking what had happened with an item that he had just made a decision on. On the third day, Rick called me in a panic, worried that we had lost the letter from his department head, congratulating him on his retirement. I reminded Rick that he had made decisions on every single piece of academic paperwork, so either he had decided to throw it away or we had saved it. The next day we found it in his filing cabinet.

Therapy would have been helpful for Rick, as a Stage 3 hoarder, but it was still optional because he would be moving in with his sister, who would help him stay clutter-free. Although Rick hadn't been diagnosed with dementia, his sister said that the signs had worsened recently and that she would continue to monitor him when they were living together. At the same time, she could really help him control his hoarding with daily reminders and incentives.

STAGE 4: AIMEE

Aimee, whose story opened this chapter, was only the second case that I'd ever worked on. We knew that her condo contained human waste and used insulin needles—two toxic substances that needed special handling—but we didn't know what else we might find. The place also had some structural damage. Late-stage hoarder houses have more potential for accidents and noxious hazards, which can put a cleanup crew at high risk for injury and sickness. With these dangers, and the legal issues about disposing of hazardous waste, a professional crew is pretty much required at this stage.

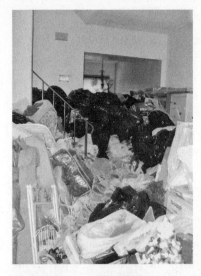

Shoes, purses, clothes, and unopened packages hid the feces and food that spilled out into the hallway from the adjacent rooms in Aimee's Stage 4 house.

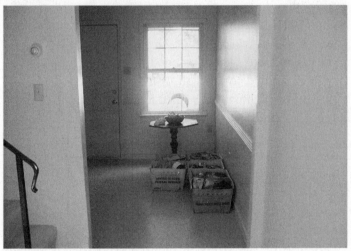

After Aimee's cleanup, there were just a few cartons of things to be taken away.

For advanced hoarders, trust is hugely important. On the first day, cleanup helpers asked Aimee for permission every time they started to work on a pile of stuff and whenever they wanted to enter a room. They asked her to look at and approve every item they threw away. It was slow going at first.

Aimee was well enough to work with us for about an hour at a time before she needed to go lie down on her bed for a rest. At first she wanted all of the workers in the same room, so that she could keep an eye on them, and she asked that the cleaning stop when she took a break. After a few days, she trusted the crew enough to allow a team to work independently in the bedroom while she stayed with the main crew in the kitchen. Everyone kept working during her breaks.

She realized that the cleaning crew wasn't going to do anything behind her back, and she knew that they were searching for important items, which included tax documents, checks, and her mother's pearl necklace. Aimee knew exactly where the necklace was. She pointed to a pile in the bathroom—clothing, towels, and newspaper, all soaking wet and moldy from the leaky sink. The next day the crew found it within two inches of where Aimee said it was, still in its original box, in perfect condition.

Aimee wanted to keep all of her purses and shoes, and most of her clothing. I reminded her of her goal—to stay in her house—and that she could either keep all her clothing *or* keep her house. So together we chose a closet just for her shoes and purses, and that space would set the limit of her hoarding. She was allowed to keep as many clothing and accessory items as she could fit into that closet, and no more. Because Aimee was learning to set her own limits, she was more agreeable when it came to making choices.

Because of the stress, a late-stage hoarder is usually unable to clean for more than a day or two. With Aimee, we scheduled two days of cleaning followed by an off day. We took her trash to the dump each day so that she wouldn't go back and pull items out of the Dumpster at night (a common hoarder problem). But Aimee's main issue was that during her non-cleaning days, she would go through her "maybe" pile and move a lot to her "keep" section. Every time the crew returned, they had to spend half a day redoing that work.

The later the hoarding stage, the more team members are usually involved to cope with the physical and emotional issues. Aimee's team included a social worker, a building inspector, and six cleanup helpers. Her cleanup took three months, with lots of days off.

The big challenge with Aimee was her emotional attachment to much of her stuff. Her "keep" items consisted mostly of things that had belonged to her late mother, who had been her closest friend and a major source of support during a difficult divorce from an abusive man. Aimee came to realize that the trauma of losing her mother had, in fact, triggered her hoarding.

Aimee's self-image had become extremely poor. It was particularly hard for her to recognize the glamorous model that she once had been. But the cleaning was an opportunity to build a new, positive attitude. One day, one of the cleanup guys found a magazine with a gorgeous, much younger Aimee on the cover. He knew it was Aimee, but he asked her who the "hot babe" was, to encourage her to embrace her former beautiful non-hoarder self. Aimee blushed and smiled; as if that was the first time she had received a compliment from a man in years. After weeks of positive reinforcement about her appearance and decision-making ability, Aimee's behavior changed. She began to smile, share stories, and became much more confident and relaxed. She began to remember her old self, before hoarding, and she enjoyed rediscovering that person.

STAGE 5: MARGARET

Margaret had been hoarding so many years that her possessions had started to decompose at the bottom of her five-foot piles. Everything in her double-wide trailer home was either broken, rotting, or chewed or peed on by the fifty or so dogs that had free run of the place. There was extensive water damage from broken pipes, with walls and ceilings split and falling down in spots. The house stank, it was hot, and the air was thick with dust. Cobwebs waved from the ceiling and flies buzzed at all of the windows.

In the kitchen, spoiled food stank up the refrigerator, and dirty dishes were molding in the sink. Cockroaches scattered whenever items were moved. The narrow walkways between the piles were swimming in a thick brown muck that actually sucked one of Margaret's clogs off her foot as she walked through the kitchen on cleanup day. She ignored it and kept walking.

In this house the hoarding had been going on for so long that everything was rotting, even the building. Once her house was condemned, Margaret moved in with one of her adult daughters who lived nearby. On cleaning day, Margaret's daughter drove her to the house to meet the cleaning crew, building inspector, animal control officer, and social worker.

With a cleanup this aggressive, it's mostly about damage control, because this stage of hoarder house will never be perfect. The building inspector told Margaret that we might get the house clean only to discover that it wasn't salvageable and had to be bulldozed. Animal control warned Margaret that the house had to pass inspection for some of her dogs to be returned.

It was hard for Margaret to say good-bye to her pets, because some of them she would never see again. In fact, getting the house clean enough for animal control to return six of the dogs became her main goal, and it motivated her through a cleanup that she really had no desire to do.

The dogs aside, the main problem for Margaret was accepting the trash in the house for what it was: just junk.

The dogs and that stuff were all that Margaret had. Most of her friends and family had abandoned her and she truly looked to the things in her house as friends. As soon as the crew started touching empty food wrappers in the kitchen and asking her if they could throw them away, Margaret's anxiety level skyrocketed and she got angry. She grabbed an empty toilet paper roll out of a worker's hands and put it in her sweater pocket, yelling at him not to handle her things. Every item they touched provoked an equally angry reaction.

I kept calm, reminded Margaret that her goal was to get her pets back, and offered to hold the trash bag open and let her choose what to throw away. This was slowgoing because Margaret didn't want to part with anything. Each item she touched had an argument attached to it about why she needed to keep it. Every time Margaret actually put an item in the bag, I congratulated her on making a really difficult move toward helping her pets. Then I told her that she only had the crew for five days, and we had to speed up the work if we were going to reach her goal.

Margaret took a day and a half to make it through the kitchen, but then the crew hit an unexpected snag. As we started cleaning out the mudroom, the crew found a massive rat's nest, nearly eight feet wide and two feet tall. We halted the cleanup until pest control could come the next day and check for rats. Fortunately, the rats were long gone and they hadn't left much damage behind except for the giant nest.

Because advanced hoarder houses always have surprises like this, the cleanup plan needs to accommodate the occasional setback and added expense. It is not at all unusual to uncover termite damage, feces, dead animals, and cracks in the foundations in a Stage 5 hoarder house.

Like Aimee, Margaret had to take frequent breaks, mostly due to the mental exhaustion of working in a constant state of anxiety and anger. She would blow up and then need to walk away to calm down. Stage 4 and 5 hoarding cleanups are massive—both physically and emotionally. Margaret had to make decisions about her possessions for the first time in more than ten years, and at her age learning a new skill was a big challenge.

The crew needed breaks too. The house was hot and the air was bad. They were working in oppressive conditions, dressed in long pants and long-sleeve shirts, with gloves, respirators, and Tyvek protective suits.

We spent five days on Margaret's house, during which time we gave her constant encouragement. By the end of the job, the only things that we were able to salvage were two bed frames, a microwave with the door held closed by duct tape, a scratched kitchen table, a few wobbly wooden chairs, and some clothing. We scrubbed everything, but the floors and walls were permanently dirty. We replaced the missing and broken ceiling tiles (which made some white and some brown), and Margaret planned to have her son-in-law fix the holes in her drywall. The floors were gouged, uneven, and permanently stained with urine, and the bottom halves of most of the doors were still missing because they had been chewed up by the dogs. The windows were dirty and there were no curtains. Her daughter planned to take her shopping to buy some new furniture and linens. Although Margaret was still angry about the cleanup and would never admit it, this was success.

THE CLEANUP PLAN

No matter how large or small the team, it's important that everyone shares the same vision and goals, especially the hoarder. The written plan, developed beforehand, gives everyone something to refer to if things get tense or arguments break out. It also gives the hoarder a black-and-white reminder of what everyone agreed to. When the pressure is on and a hoarder is panicking, everyone can take a step back, calm down, and refer to the plan to get back on track.

Because cleanups are unpredictable, plans need to be flexible to account for surprises like finding structural damage in a house, or the realization that meeting a predetermined deadline will be impossible. But everyone should agree *together* on changes and work on implementing the updated plan.

▶ Team Members

Even if it's a small team, take the time to introduce everyone. Especially with extreme hoarding jobs, not all of the team members may be present at the outset. But the team leader should, at the least, have a list of everyone who will be involved. Knowing the players is most important for anxious hoarders whose suspicions may still be high at this early stage of the cleanup.

This is also a good time to divide up the job and decide who will be working on what part of the cleanup. The team leader should remind everyone that the hoarder is the boss, which is one more way to reinforce trust throughout the cleanup. Any team members who come later in the process should identify themselves to the hoarder so that the hoarder knows they belong there and aren't just curious onlookers.

Someone should always be designated to be the hoarder's advocate. This is a particularly challenging job and may fall to the person who knows the hoarder well, has the hoarder's confidence, and can empathetically represent his or her interests.

Team Colors

EVEN WITH A team of all volunteers, we like to make sure everyone wears the same color shirts to show uniformity. While reinforcing the "team" concept for the cleanup crew and the hoarder, the shirts also represent a big step for the hoarder, who has not been a part of any group in a long time. Hoarders who work hard that first day earn a Clutter Cleaner T-shirt, making them part of our crew. We don't hand out freebies; they only get the shirt when they give 100 percent effort.

▶ Dates and Scheduling

Most of the hoarders with whom I work try to cancel their cleanup at least once. Even when they are finally committed to the big day, I often find them unprepared. The hoarder may delay the start in order to "tidy up" a bit before the crew enters the house. And it is the job of the designated point person, or team leader, to remind the hoarder that they are there to work on the cleanup *together*.

Advanced hoarders have often been evicted from a condemned property and are living elsewhere. They often arrive late for the cleanup: Sometimes they are genuinely running behind, but I've figured out that some hoarders are testing to see if they really have control of the situation. They need to see that the crew waits for them to begin a cleanup. Starting without the hoarder being present, or getting angry because a hoarder is late, just reinforces the hoarder's mistrust. Without trust, the cleanup will go straight downhill.

I start each cleanup day with a meeting of everyone on the team who will be involved that day. Even if the team is just the hoarder and a helper, the meeting reinforces the message that this cleanup is serious and confirms that the hoarder isn't in this alone. We recap the previous day's accomplishments, lay out the new day's plan, and answer any questions.

▶ **Goals and Expectations**

"Our goal here today is for Margaret to clean her house up and get her dogs back."

Each day may start with a meeting, but more important, it begins with a reminder of the goals and expectations to which everyone has agreed. Starting on a positive and supportive note reminds hoarders that although they may be feeling anxious, they have chosen to take this action to get a result that is meaningful to them: to keep their house, get their kids or pets back, be able to invite friends over, or reconnect with their family.

This is also a good time to review the schedule and logistics for the cleaning crew, which rooms to tackle first, and what will happen if we fall behind the schedule. We also have to remind ourselves of deadlines that have been imposed, such as those enforced by city or county officials or health and welfare services. And don't hesitate to remind everyone not only of the positive goals but also of the negative consequences—fines, loss of the home, or other unfortunate outcomes.

Timeline goals are what I call "we" goals: The entire team, not just the hoarder, takes responsibility for cleaning the house in the time allotted. If that deadline has to be extended, while it's often 100 percent the hoarder's fault, it is better to take responsibility as a team. Hoarders who understand that they are not alone in the process are more likely to succeed.

During the cleanup, the team will want to refer to the life goal frequently, to keep the hoarder on track. Whenever a hoarder starts to waffle, drag his or her feet, or hang on to too many items, it's time to remind the hoarder of the overall goals, and what must be done to reach them.

▶ Homework

To get a good sense of realistic goals, it's critical to find out what hoarders are able to do on their own. During the cleanup, we roll out the idea of "homework," giving the hoarder a small task to complete overnight, maybe sorting through one box, or taking out three bags of trash. If the hoarder is able to follow through on this homework, that individual probably has enough self-discipline to work with checklists after the cleaning is done. If a hoarder doesn't respond to homework, then the hoarder's issues are probably deep enough to require serious support in the form of therapy, an organizer, or a cleaning helper before the hoarder can work through a checklist alone.

Each hoarder should have different homework that's tailored to that hoarder's particular issues. No matter what the homework, every hoarder needs to do those assignments every night, both during the cleaning and afterward, just like in school. The point of homework is to build the discipline of doing something to stay clean every single day.

▶ The Fire List

All hoarders have several key items that they want to locate and keep. Rick was looking for his house deed and employment letters. Daisy knew she had some savings bonds in her house. Aimee wanted to find her mother's pearls. Margaret hoped we could find her hearing aid and a missing pair of glasses.

Hoarders should write down everything they would want to keep if there was a fire, limiting the list to the front of one piece of paper. While we don't want to add to hoarders' anxiety, we do actually make them go through the exercise of trying to find and gather the items on the fire list in two minutes—the time they would have if the house was on fire. This process proves to hoarders that they can't actually find important items in that limited time frame. It also helps hoarders be selective in limiting the number of items. Making a list helps the hoarder learn and internalize organizational skills instead of just being told what and how to do something by family or friends.

Whatever the items, no matter how silly they may sound, they are gold to the hoarder. Finding them proves to the hoarder that the cleanup is effective and reinforces the hoarder's trust. Usually a hoarder knows roughly (sometimes exactly) where the items are, so everyone should be made aware not only of what's on the list but any clues that the hoarder provides as to their whereabouts. (We print copies of the fire list and tape it to the walls in every room, or make sure every team member has a copy.)

Creating a fire list on the first day—and reviewing it each day during the job—not only makes it more likely you'll find the items, but also confirms to the hoarder that his or her wishes are being taken very seriously. The hoarder will realize that the entire team is there to find what the hoarder feels is important. When those items are uncovered, stop the cleanup and celebrate! Make sure everyone shares the feeling of success, because moments like that can get a team through a tough job.

▶ Process and Logistics

Everyone needs to know what the order of work will be—where the work will begin, what priorities have been set, how long everyone will be working, and so on. The logistics of the cleanup should be spelled out clearly, such as where items will be staged, where trash will be piled, and which door to use to enter and exit the house.

The Legacy Cleanup

WHEN JIM DIED, he left behind a house full of hoarded paperwork and collectibles for his three adult children to clean up. The kids were prepared—they knew the house was bad. Jim, who had been a well-educated preacher, had spent his life collecting memorabilia and historical collectibles from black history.

Jim's children had tried on occasion to get their father to clean, but they respected him too much to start a fight. His house, although eight of the ten rooms were filled, was still safe. And up until his death he had been pretty self-sufficient, even after his wife had died and cleaning was the least of his concerns.

Under the circumstances, Jim's family decided to leave him alone, but they knew that when their father died they'd have to clean and sell the house. In preparation for that eventuality, they asked their father if there were specific things that he would like the children—or anyone else, for that matter—to have. It was sort of an informal part of his will and the children assured Jim that they'd respect his wishes.

After Jim passed away, his sons and daughter went through a mourning period. Because they couldn't handle the emotions of the cleanup on top of the loss in their family, they closed up the house and let it sit for about a year. Had they jumped into cleaning right away, it would have been tempting to keep a lot of Jim's things, especially because so many of them were actually valuable historical items. This is one way I see hoarding passed from generation to generation.

For Jim's family, the waiting period turned out to be a good thing, because after a year had passed they weren't as emotional, and they were willing to let more items go. First, they finalized the cleanup plan. Then they divided up the items that Jim had already designated to go to certain family members. For the rest, they drew straws and took turns choosing additional things they wanted to keep. After that, they organized a big yard sale. For them, that was almost like a big party. They had all grown up in that house, and the neighbors came by to reconnect and pick up a few mementos.

The sorting, cleaning, and yard sale could have been really stressful, because a legacy cleanup presents some unique challenges. Without the hoarder present, there's no one to give the cleaning crew clues as to where valuables may be hidden (which is often the case with hoarders). And unless there's a single surviving family member who's been designated to be in charge, things can get dicey if the family starts squabbling over stuff. On top of this, the emotional issues for family members who've lost a loved one need to be considered.

A family doing a legacy cleanup has to agree on what the goal is and how to get there. The planning process can take longer and be more contentious without the hoarder, since the overall purpose isn't always clear. One family member might want to sell the house, another might want to live there, and yet another might not be ready for cleaning and just want to wait. This kind of cleanup runs more smoothly the more time a family puts into assessing and creating a careful and equitable plan.

Team members need to know if any parts of the house aren't being cleaned or if there are rooms off-limits, either for safety or structural reasons, or for privacy issues. And everyone needs to know where the hoarder will be working, so they can find that person to ask questions.

Any cost issues are usually private, between family members and the hoarder, or discussed with whoever is paying the bill. The actual numbers may be confidential, but it is helpful for members of the team to be aware that some decisions may be determined by the cost. Rick, for example, initially wanted to shred his paperwork, but when the estimate was over $20,000, he decided to just have it hauled to the dump for recycling. The team didn't need to know the price, but they did need to know about the change in plan.

As with every aspect of the cleanup, reviewing the plan logistics with the hoarder as well as with the team in advance will create trust and lower the likelihood of drama as the cleaning unfolds.

DEALING WITH HOARDER REACTIONS

No cleanup will work unless everyone is aware of the many emotional and psychological issues that can delay or derail even the best-laid plan. I knew, for example, that Aimee felt really anxious about anyone entering her bedroom, so I made sure the team respected that and asked her permission each time someone went in.

If a hoarder has specific mental issues and is open about discussing them, then early in the cleanup is a good time to mention it. Say the cleanup is for an OCD hoarder who has to touch every item. The plan should try to build that awareness in as much as possible. The team leader can remind everyone, including the hoarder, that although the OCD is a legitimate issue, the hoarder might need to work on giving up some control if the job is to get done by the deadline. The team leader should use positive reinforcement, such as saying, "Lucy had a really tough day yesterday; we want to acknowledge that she made some hard decisions. Great job, Lucy."

As the cleanup progresses, the morning meetings provide a good opportunity to give the hoarder lots of encouragement and praise for his or her participation, especially in front of family members. Cleaning is challenging, and hoarders are working on new skills as they go through it. Positive feedback helps reinforce that.

Every hoarder has issues, even if it's a Stage 1 hoarder like Brad, who was attached to his computer stash. Going over those issues will alert team members to possible behaviors that could pop up during the cleaning.

Once the cleaning begins in earnest, many of the underlying psychological and emotional issues that plague a hoarder may surface in unexpected ways, with lots of drama and probably some panic. During cleanup, helpers are not only stripping hoarders of their possessions, but also removing a comforting behavior that has made up for a lot of hurt.

There's no such thing as too much praise for a hoarder who is trying to de-clutter. Extreme hoarders have felt like failures for years, maybe decades, and it may take a while for them to accept the praise. The solution is to pour it on—not false praise, but sincere acknowledgment for the hard work they are doing. Appreciation is something everyone wants in life, and it's no different for a hoarder. Ironically, that need for appreciation is something that has usually fueled the hoarding.

A hoarder's behavior during a cleanup is driven by a sometimes fragile emotional state that is best navigated with social workers, therapists, or clergy. But family members can also get on board and really help once they know what the process is likely to dredge up.

► Freaking Out

Being clean scared Aimee. She didn't know where anything was in her newly cleaned rooms. Suddenly, she was losing control of the stuff that she'd kept cataloged in her brain. Every evening after the cleaners left, we learned, Aimee would become irrational and start looking for things that randomly came to mind. Because many of these things had already been moved or discarded, when she couldn't find them, she called me. Realizing what Aimee was going through, I made her daily call a part of her process. I told her that while I fully expected her to call me, she had to do so before 9:00 p.m. This arrangement allowed her to accept and own her behavior, but also put some limits on it.

The freak-out is actually a good sign. Many hoarders have literally built a wall of trash around themselves to mentally and physically protect them from the real world. A cleanup crew is tearing down this wall of protection. A hoarder who shows no emotions at all is probably not processing the cleanup seriously. Chances are that the house will be full again very soon.

► Stonewalling

At first, Nika, a Stage 3 clothes hoarder, didn't engage in the cleaning process at all. She sat like a lump on a pile of clothing in the living room and wouldn't even talk to the cleaning crew. I could see that she was refusing to face the fear and anxiety of the cleaning. She was retreating away from reality. So I pushed over one of her piles.

It was an eight-foot stack of clothing and shoes, and I "accidentally" hit it with my hip, hard. When it came tumbling down, Nika lost her cool. She jumped up to grab her things and start piling them back up, all the while yelling at me to quit messing with her stuff.

My goal is always to get a hoarder engaged in a positive way, but if that doesn't happen then I'll accept their anger. After my little accident, Nika realized that working *with* us was the only way to protect her valuables, and she joined in the cleanup. Knocking over her beloved pile may not have been a textbook psychological move, but it did get Nika to do things she hadn't done in years: engage, take control, and make decisions.

The hoarder has usually been avoiding emotions for so long that getting back in touch with them is scary and painful. We want hoarders to reconnect with their emotions, and expressing anger is often the first step toward that goal. Anger is a powerful emotion, but it is often better to vent it than to succumb to a more debilitating and paralyzing emotion, like grief or fear.

Being the brunt of a hoarder's flash of anger can be scary and upsetting, but remember that the hoarder is actually angry at himself or herself. Hoarders may not even realize it, but by yelling at those around them, they are actually venting their frustration with having let their life become so out of control.

▶ **Lashing Out**

Some hoarders choose to be alone because they have lost someone in the past. On the surface it looks like a hoarder wants to be alone, but the truth is the hoarder doesn't want to get close to someone else and risk another loss or death. I see this often in older women, like Margaret, who put on a "tough" persona. They'll start cussing and fighting and calling me bad names right away. I call this reaction "the rattlesnake."

Fighting like this has kept the rattlesnake isolated and safe from contact, so she tries it again with the cleaning crew. To the hoarder, getting rid of people is much easier than the risk of attaching to them. From our experience, it appears that the more anger a hoarder releases during a cleanup, the deeper the hoarder's fear and hurt. It's critical to stick with the cleaning so hoarders realize that not everyone abandons them.

When a "rattlesnake" hoarder starts yelling, she is trying to suck the cleaning crew into a negative interaction. She is doing what has always worked in the past—get angry, yell, and make people leave. She's testing us.

It's the cleaning team's job to stay positive and not get sucked into that game. The crew might need to step outside and take frequent breaks. Even if the hoarder is obviously the one who needs to take five, I always say it's me. I tell her that she's doing great and may not need it, but I'm exhausted and need a quick break. Then I go out and take some deep breaths or vent to one of the other team members (out of the hoarder's earshot, of course).

Sometimes I even joke about it. When a rattlesnake lashes out and starts yelling at me, I will say, "Hey, there's no time for flirting. Let's get back to work." The hoarder is expecting me to get pissed, so a joke totally shakes up the dynamic.

▶ Pushing for Control

Aimee, the former model, was a control freak during the cleanup phase. She had to touch or look at every single item, even five-year-old old junk mail and plastic shopping bags, which can be frustrating for a cleanup crew. But when Aimee came to understand that she was the one who would decide what to throw away and what to save, she realized that she did, indeed, have power over her situation.

Aimee had been called a slob and a loser for years. To be able to keep her house, she had to believe that she could be a clutter-free winner. And the only way she could learn that about herself was to take control and make the right choices on her own.

When a hoarder starts pushing for control, that's something a helper should celebrate. It may slow down the cleanup process, but it can empower a hoarder to take control of other parts of his or her life.

It is also possible for a cleanup organizer to control the hoarder's control. One way to position this is to give the hoarder a choice between two options, "You are in control. Do you want us to throw away item A or item B?" The hoarder controls which item goes, but the crew has controlled the process and the options. A hoarder should focus on letting go, so whenever possible, it's important to phrase options as "donate" or "trash" rather than "keep."

During the cleanup, Aimee got a lot of praise about her ability to make good choices. At first she didn't respond to positive reinforcement, but by the end of the cleanup she was clearly making choices to hear the praise from the cleaning crew and her daughter.

▶ **Expressing Anxiety**

Jackson, the Blondie hoarder, had a lot of anxiety. Over the phone he assured me that his house was worse than I could even imagine. I insisted that I had seen truly awful houses, and besides I didn't really care about the state of the house, I cared about him as a person. Jackson also got very anxious during and even after the cleanup.

When cleaning starts, hoarders tend to pick up and clutch items in their hands without putting them down. Pretty soon their arms and pockets start to fill up like they are a squirrel storing for the winter. They talk very fast and won't look people in the eye. These are sure signs that anxiety is taking over. Someone having an anxiety attack simply can't function.

Dealing with anxiety is not necessarily the job of the cleanup crew, which is why it's essential to have a trusted and empathetic advocate on call—a therapist, social worker, or clergyman—who is not involved in the physical cleanup. Depending on the severity of the hoarder's anxiety, the cleanup may be halted briefly, or for a longer time if other professional and emotional support is needed.

Trying to power through the cleaning process with a hoarder having an anxiety attack will only make it worse. Ignoring these emotions and not listening to the hoarder could cause major issues down the road for the cleaning and the relationship.

▶ Retreating into Denial

Most hoarders are in denial at some level. Even hoarders who finally seem ready to clean up may head right into denial once the process begins. That's where Thalia went. Even before she locked herself in her car and tried to swallow the pills, Thalia was rationalizing everything. She talked about how all of her things had importance, her mess wasn't that bad, and she wasn't even a hoarder.

Unlike the other potential responses, *denial is a dealbreaker*. I'll clean up a house full of anxiety any day of the week, but a house full of denial will stay full. When I hear denial from a hoarder, I stop everything and we talk. Often the hoarder will admit to being scared and that the process is hard. I will assure the hoarder that I respect that honesty and the fact that he or she is willing to take on such a difficult challenge. On some jobs that same conversation has been repeated every day.

I had planned to give Thalia two days to come around and hopefully face her issues. I frequently reminded her that when my crew first came on she had already acknowledged that her hoarding was a problem. I asked her how that had changed. I was waiting for the moment when she would admit that she needed to stop hoarding. Most of the hoarders I work with eventually get there, but Thalia never did.

When a hoarder like Thalia keeps insisting that everything is fine, then the cleanup is probably premature. When I hear denial, I don't get angry, because I've come to understand that it's an integral part of a hoarder's mental process. But I also don't waste my time trying to clean up a house that I know will be full again in six months.

▶ Dealing with Grief

Not every hoarder is grieving from a recent loss, but some have had deaths or divorces that they are still processing. Others grieve the loss of their stuff. This is normal, and helpers have a great opportunity to support a hoarder who needs to work through grief and let it go.

When I started cleaning houses for a living, my first paying customer was my grandmother. She hired me to help clean out her basement, which was full of gardening equipment, tools, and boxes of my late grandfather's things. My grandmother was not a hoarder; we were just trying to help each other out.

While I simply wanted to get the job done, about halfway through, I realized that she was struggling emotionally. She wasn't ready yet to let my grandfather's things go. Instead, she wanted to spend time enjoying the happy memories those things brought up.

I had been volunteering for about two years at Comfort Zone Camp, a camp for bereaved children in Richmond, Virginia. As part of our counselor training, they taught us some techniques for encouraging kids to talk about their grief. When I saw that my grandmother was deep in that same grieving place, I decided to use some of the techniques I had learned with the kids.

So, instead of asking why she was holding on to some old golf bag, I asked her what it brought to mind. She started telling me stories about my grandfather, and then finally she said, "I guess we don't need that anymore. We can let it go." I could see her physically release her grief. And when she let that go, she could also release his possessions.

I've learned that for hoarders, every cleanup is a grieving process. We are asking them to say good-bye to items that are heavy with memories—some wonderful, some painful. But all are important and deserve respect. A hoarder finds safety in the hoard, in the stacks and piles, and he or she will grieve over the loss of those items when they are gone. The week after the house cleaning is usually the worst. Instead of being happy and enjoying the new space, hoarders go through a difficult process. They miss their possessions, which were their closest friends for years.

WHERE HOARDER STUFF GOES

A hoarder's things may look like trash to someone helping with a cleanup, but the hoarder usually has plans for those items. During a cleanup, the crew's job is to implement those plans. That may mean making phone calls to find donation sites, talking to auction houses about selling items, or listing things on eBay. Disposing of a hoarder's things can take as much time as the cleanup itself.

During the course of our cleanups we regularly have to handle anything from dead animals to diapers filled with human waste, junk cars to old containers of pesticides, insulin needles to bloodstained clothing. None of this can be simply bagged and tossed at the dump, as it requires special handling. Not only is it the law, but a lot of this stuff is toxic and can cause serious injury if it's not disposed of correctly.

And that's to say nothing of live animals, pests, and vermin, which also require special attention.

▶ Dumping

The Environmental Protection Agency's website lists hazardous waste that must be disposed of by approved methods and facilities. (See the resources section at the back of this book for contact information.) During a cleanup, it is best to put suspected toxic items to the side, make a list, and then contact the EPA or other agency to determine how best to handle each type of material.

For example, used needles have to be taken to a medical waste facility, where they are incinerated. A biohazard like human feces must go there too, as does anything with blood on it. As human waste sits, it develops deadly microbes, bacteria, and viruses. Flies spread those around, so a house where human waste is only in one room may still have e-coli present in other parts of the house. The hoarder may have been living in the house for years, but that doesn't make it safe. Chemicals, paints, paint thinners, and batteries also require special handling. A local dump should either have special days for hazardous waste drop-off or know of a nearby site that takes it.

With any of these materials, cleanup crews should be fully protected by masks, Tyvek suits, and heavy gloves. The fumes alone can sometimes be deadly or can burn human skin. Wearing protective gear may feel awkward when the hoarder is walking around the house in normal clothes, but nobody knows what hidden ailments the hoarder has developed. And it's impossible to predict someone's reaction to a chemical—one person might be fine, another might have a life-threatening reaction. It's not worth the risk.

Dead pets must be either cremated by a certified facility or buried (some localities no longer allow burials so check local regulations). Dead pests, like mice, must be handled by pest control experts, who know how to protect against the diseases their bodies and feces carry. Mice and rats can eat all kinds of toxins and survive to litter those chemicals around the house in their waste, which makes them extra dangerous. A rule of thumb that we use is that for every live mouse seen in the house, there are ten more in the walls.

Old cars can be dangerous because of the oils, antifreeze, and gasoline that might still be inside. The safest disposal method is to call a wrecker or tow truck to haul away the vehicle, and the driver will usually pay something for it because the car can be sold for scrap metal value. When in doubt about whether or not something is hazardous, or how to dispose of it, call the EPA and ask.

▶ Donating

Hoarders often have an easier time parting with items when they know they will go to good use. Brad and Ellen donated their boxed and canned food to a local food bank. Household items can go to whatever donation sites the hoarder cares about and wants to support. Charities and churches may decline certain items, so be prepared with alternatives.

For useful household items, we usually recommend a local battered women's shelter because they help people who are truly in immediate need. Families often arrive there empty-handed and can use bedding, clothing, toiletries, and small appliances. Larger donation sites, like Goodwill, often sell the bulk of their items to third world countries.

An organization such as the Salvation Army will often pick up donations quickly. People feel good about helping other people, and hoarders are no different. They are often motivated to give something away if they have an emotional connection with the charity, and it's reassuring to know that their things will be well used.

Some hoarders hang on to family mementos, intending to pass them to future generations. Here, the hoarder needs to prove that the family member actually wants the item. Does the hoarder's niece really want her aunt's costume jewelry? This is another opportunity for a hoarder reality check. If the family member doesn't care, then there is no reason to save the item.

I see a lot of hoarders saving soda bottle tops because they've read somewhere that a child in the hospital needs them to raise money for some type of surgery or organ transplant. I don't know if the story is an urban legend or not, but I do know that many hoarders have been saving these bottle tops for years, by which point, little Timmy is either a dad with his own kids or has passed on. Either way, Timmy doesn't need those bottle tops anymore.

▶ Selling

Nika was a clothes hoarder extraordinaire, and a lot of her items had never been worn. She had ordered most of the clothes from a television shopping channel, and a lot of things were still in the original packaging. Nika was convinced that she was going to make a fortune selling her clothing. In Nika's mind, the clothing was worth what she paid for it. She expected to earn all that back.

Unfortunately, that's rare. Most hoarders are convinced their collections are valuable, but usually what they have just isn't collectible. Even if there is a market for the items, the price isn't anywhere near what the hoarder paid, and often the value is so low that it's not even worth the trouble to sell the stuff.

Nika thought she could sell her clothing in a consignment store. But the first store she visited rejected more than half of what she brought in (too out-of-style, or the label wasn't impressive enough), and for the rest they offered Nika pennies on the dollar. She eventually took what was offered and donated the rest of the clothes.

Some collectibles and antiques have real value, but there's almost always a huge difference between what the hoarder paid (or thinks something is worth) and what someone else is willing to pay. The reality is that any item is only worth what someone will pay for it.

If the items are useful, consider a yard sale or an auction house. These options work particularly well for shopping hoarders, who often have a big collection of new items still in the boxes. An auction house will only get a small percentage of the new price of the item, but it's better than nothing.

I often hear hoarders tell me that they are going to sell an item on eBay. I ask if they have ever sold an item online, and most of them acknowledge that they do not even have a working computer. The truth is that they know they have blown a lot of money on their collection and they are hoping to get some back. If money is not an issue, encourage donation. If money is an issue, go with the auction houses. Selling items one by one at a place like eBay is not realistic and can lead to more hoarding and buying online.

Unfortunately, selling items doesn't mean they're gone. Thalia, a television shopping network addict, sent most of her collectibles to an auction house. The day of the auction, Thalia was in the front row, tearfully bidding to buy back all of her items. Thalia proves that a successful cleanup doesn't end with a clean house. A hoarder has to *stay* clean, which means working day after day on new life skills, and replacing the hoarding behavior with something fulfilling.

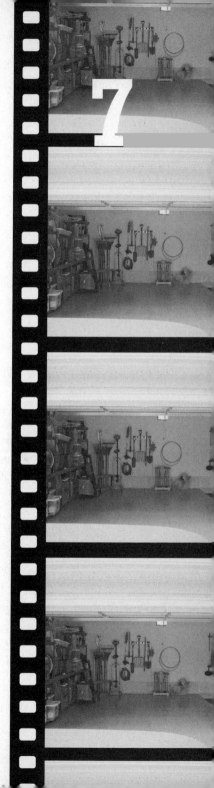

7

STAYING
CLEAN

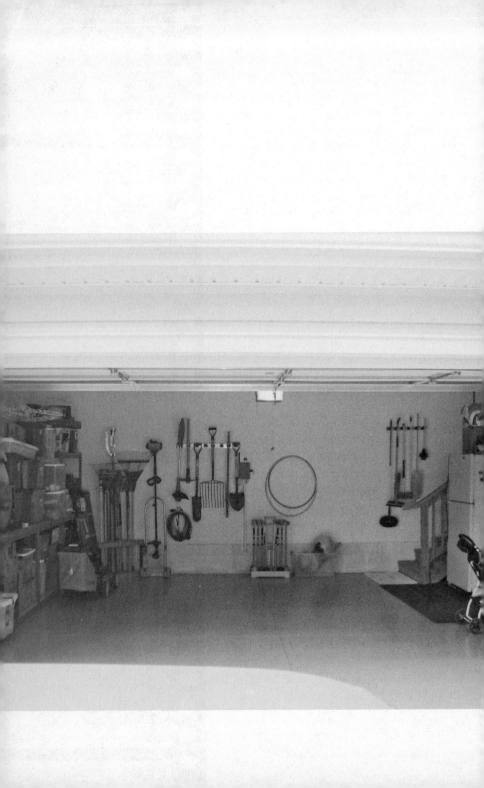

Li's large, hundred-year-old farmhouse and barn in rural Connecticut were filled with top-quality clothing and appliances. There was no trash.

With her children grown and living away when her husband died, Li slipped completely out of control as she took to shopping to ease her loneliness. When her daughter, Sunny, called me, she said that the house had been cluttered when they were growing up, but now it was so bad that Li was pretty well confined to living in the kitchen and its adjoining bathroom.

Li was unusual in that she didn't look like a stereotypical hoarder. Now in her early eighties, she appeared to be thirty years younger. She was always well turned out in designer clothes, nicely made up, and well groomed. That she still cared about her looks seemed to be a sign that she might care enough to want a tidy house.

Li's children had tried to get her to clean up for years, but she fought it and just kept shopping. Finally, Sunny put together a carefully researched "business plan" outlining the advantages of de-cluttering the house, and begged her mother to try a single day of cleaning. If she didn't like that, Sunny assured her she would send the crew away.

Li was an old-school parent, very authoritarian and always wanting to be in charge, so nobody knew what to expect when our crew of ten came into the house to handle her possessions.

Fortunately, Li was ready to get it done. Because her family had let *her* make the decision and presented her with a plan that made sense to her, Li stayed engaged in the process, realizing the benefits to having a clean house. After meeting the crew briefly, she trusted her children enough to go and stay at one of their houses while the work was being done.

On that first day, at the bottom of a six-foot pile of kitchen appliances and boxes of food, the crew found $40,000 worth of savings bonds. Sunny called to tell Li the exciting news, and although she was still anxious, that convinced her to continue with the cleanup. Li had thought the bonds were expired, and we were happy to explain the difference between expiration and maturity.

We spent five days cleaning and ended up loading two eighteen-wheeler trucks full of items to donate to the nearby shelter.

After the cleanup, the house looked pretty good. The downstairs carpet needed to be replaced and the walls needed painting. But the hundred-year-old structure was sturdy enough that it had withstood a decade of hoarding without any serious damage.

Li was delighted with her new, empty house. She had actually forgotten how huge the house was. Until the cleanup, her hoarding had become the only topic of discussion between Li and her daughters, and none of them wanted that to continue. After the cleanup, the time Li spent with her family was so much happier—and motivated her to stay clean.

Therapy is a critical part of staying clean for advanced hoarders, and fortunately Li was open to working with a therapist, who helped her understand the issues driving her hoarding urge and how to deal with those in a more positive way. Li started spending time with her daughters and grand-children instead of buying them things.

THE ELEMENTS OF SUCCESS

Cleaning is easy; nearly anyone can empty a hoarded house. The real challenge is helping a hoarder make the lifestyle changes needed to stay clean. The longer a hoarder has been collecting, the harder those changes are, and the more support and help the hoarder needs. An early-stage hoarder can probably get by with a few checklists and a daily tidying up. A hard-core hoarder needs family, friends, therapy, maybe an organizer, and pretty much a whole new way of living his or her life. Like any addiction, hoarding is something the hoarder will face and fight every single day, and the more support that person has, the more likely it is that he or she will be successful. From my experience with hundreds of hoarders, I've discovered that there are some elements that can determine a hoarder's best chance for success.

▶ Desire to Change

Unless the cleanup is an intervention, a hoarder's wish and intention are probably already in play, or else the hoarder wouldn't have agreed to go through the process. I knew that newlyweds Wendy and Sam, for example, were motivated to change, because when they talked about the hoarding they admitted it was a problem. Wendy said that she knew it was interfering with their relationship, and the relationship they had with their children.

By contrast, I could tell that Roxanne, the hoarder who had saved all of her adult child's baby and childhood stuff, had no desire to clean. Her intervention was instigated by a social worker, who was as concerned about Roxanne's declining health as she was about the hoarding. Besides, Roxanne was still in denial. She didn't believe that a cleanup would make her life better. For a hoarder who has no desire to change, the house may get clean through an intervention, but it won't stay that way.

Recovery is hard work. The thing that motivates a hoarder through each day is the desire to have a better life. Without that, it's just too easy to give up.

▶ Recognizing Self-Worth

Although it sounds counterintuitive, hoarders care very much what others think. But if they cared so much, and wanted a relationship so badly, they'd clean up, right? Of course, but it's not that simple. In my experience, hoarding begins with the hoarder not feeling loved or appreciated. The hoarding starts as a childlike response, akin to running away and saying, "I don't really need you!" but then watching to see if anyone follows. I see hoarding as a cry for help.

That's why I tell hoarders that they need to want to de-clutter for *themselves*, not anyone else. Not for family members who promise they will be more loving. Not for their spouses or even, sadly, for their children. Those motivations won't hold up in the long run. Hoarders have to stop making choices based on how they want others to react and just make a choice for themselves.

When hoarders allow themselves to care what other people think, they put themselves in a state of inequality. By valuing other people's opinion more highly than their own, hoarders obviously rank themselves second. This self-imposed inequality is often a catalyst for long-term failure.

By putting such importance on someone else's opinion, the hoarder is also inviting judgment into his or her life. In my experience, judgment and a perceived lack of acceptance are at the root of most hoarding. When people make the choice to not let the opinion of others hurt or sway them, then they are taking control of their life and making themselves equal to the rest of the world. In my experience, the hoarder must love himself or herself fully before the hoarder can be of value to another person.

What we've seen in hoarding is that when people care about someone else's views more than their own, they start to look for physical possessions to show others their self-worth. But people who fully love and respect themselves won't need "stuff" to prove their worth.

I'm not saying the hoarder shouldn't care about family or friends. It's the reverse—I'm actually challenging hoarders to share real relationships, and show their personality and value through conversation and emotions instead of through physical objects. Short-term success can be achieved by being motivated by what others think, but long-term success is only reached when hoarders do it for themselves.

▶ Accepting Responsibility

Janelle was someone who relished "fighting the system." By hoarding food and keeping items far after their expiration date, she was refusing to let someone else tell her what she could or could not eat. She struggled with what she saw as arbitrarily imposed restrictions on her life.

Many hoarders simply stop trying and, whether actively (like Janelle) or passively, they ignore the basic rules that we've come to expect functioning members of society to follow. Hoarders who want to get their lives back have to recognize and accept these basics, whether they involve looking after personal hygiene, having a job, respecting their neighbors, or living within a budget. Those rules seem fundamental to most people, but they can feel restrictive to a hoarder who has lived for years without them.

Perhaps one of the most significant issues for many

hoarders is the management of their finances. For most, the solution is ending the use of credit. As far as I am concerned, this should be a hard-and-fast rule, especially when people have put themselves into debt with their acquisitions or are simply living on credit because they have lost control of their finances.

After my gambling problem, I lost everything and was forced to use cash only. Although it was hard, not having credit cards was one of the best things that ever happened to me. I learned during those years to ask myself if I needed an item or just wanted it, and I also figured out how to make myself happy by *doing* something instead of *buying* something.

I encourage hoarders to ask themselves these questions whenever they are tempted to shop: Will this item make my life better? Does it help me keep my home in order? If this is a gift, does the person I am buying it for really want or need it? If I don't have enough cash for this, am I willing to wait until I do?

Living without a credit card forces people to get their financial house in order, just as they have to get their physical house in shape.

▶ No Quitting

I've always believed that a hoarder house is a house full of quitting. To make a change, the hoarder has to stop quitting and start trying. The hoarder has to want to change. I have heard hundreds of hoarders' stories, and they all start with one or more tragic events. We are all challenged in life, and sometimes challenged to the point of failure. A hoarder is someone who has responded to those challenges by giving up in one or more places in life, including battling clutter.

The worst part about quitting is that every time someone

makes that choice, it gets easier to do it again. Of course, there is a difference between quitting and making a strategic decision to stop. Stopping makes sense when someone has exhausted every ounce of effort and continuing to push forward would be emotionally or psychologically damaging. But stopping before giving 100 percent is quitting.

When hoarders quit, they are cheating their potential. Every time they quit, they are taking a shortcut and they know it. The guilt builds, which is why hoarders can't allow themselves to quit again, not even once. Quitting on small actions eventually leads to completely giving up. And completely giving up is what fills a house with junk and leaves a hoarder hopeless and feeling alone.

I am diligent and firm about the "no quitting" rule with hoarders. It's much bigger than just one quick decision not to wash the dishes one night because it's easier to sit on the couch in front of the TV. Hoarders need to learn how to make themselves do things that they don't want to do. Building that self-discipline is what will keep a hoarder clean for a lifetime.

▶ Rebuilding a Network of Family and Friends

It's one thing to have professionals on call, and pay them for their services, but perhaps the most critical engagement that a hoarder can have to ensure ongoing success is a strong network of family and friends involved in his or her welfare.

When it was time on the last day of cleaning for us to leave Katrina, the divorcée who had studied to become a lawyer, we left her with two rooms to finish on her own, full of her skin care supplies and legal paperwork. As we packed up, she kept finding extra little jobs for us to do. The crew had cleaned alongside her for several days, helping sort through her extensive legal files and divorce records. We didn't judge her, we just joked and had fun, and we all enjoyed the time in her house. By the end of the cleanup, we had become Katrina's best friends—and she didn't want us to leave.

A cleaning team may be the only people a hoarder has let into the house in years. The fact that the hoarder even lets someone inside is a huge deal. The hoarder shares personal stories and is at a vulnerable time in his or her life. By the time the cleaning is done, the team members are usually the closest, most trusted contacts the hoarder has in the outside world.

Not wanting us to leave is a positive thing! It means the hoarder is enjoying relationships and rediscovering the ability to connect with other people. A hoarder's social skills are often rusty. It can be awkward at first because sometimes a hoarder has forgotten how to have relationships. Family and friends need to be very tolerant and forgiving as they help direct this positive impulse back out into the world.

I always suggest planning something social for when the cleaning is done. For example, one of Aimee's goals was to invite friends into her home. We set a date about six months from the cleaning start date for her to have a party, which gave her a realistic deadline for getting the house cleaned up and keeping it clean after we left. The party date was at the same time as the season finale of the television show *Sex and the City*, so Aimee decided to invite four girlfriends from her past to watch the show.

It went really well. It was the first time Aimee had had people in the house in eight years, and she was thrilled that the visit wasn't about hoarding, or shame, or explaining and defending her mess. Instead, it was about friends enjoying one another's company and about her being able to offer hospitality to her guests. Her friends were also glad just to see her again. They kept commenting on how great it was to have her back in their lives. This experience started Aimee on a positive path toward a social future. Aimee had really bonded with the cleaning crew, and in fact, she is still one of my favorite people in the world. She is one of the first people I call on Christmas morning.

Family members are usually the natural first connection for a hoarder to make. They can point a hoarder toward a wider social circle that can include friends, support groups, classes, work, volunteering, or hobbies and pastimes. Aimee's friends from a decade earlier returned to her life and rallied to support her after the cleanup, proving that true friendship will still be there for a hoarder when he or she decides to reconnect.

▶ Undergoing Therapy

No matter how intent a person may be, or how willing to take responsibility for his or her actions, sometimes it is simply impossible to do it alone. Without professional follow-up therapy, up to 85 percent of serious hoarders will go right back into the behavior. Even with therapy, I see up to half of late-stage hoarders slip back into it.

Li talked about her shopping compulsion with a therapist who specialized in obsessive-compulsive behavior and hoarding. What she really worked on were the issues that were driving her shopping. Her therapist helped her see why she felt the need to have designer clothes, a Mercedes, and expensive jewelry. Li realized that she had issues from being an immigrant with minimal education who initially had to raise her children in a tiny house in a run-down neighborhood. Every time Li bought herself a designer purse or a pair of earrings, or an expensive gift for a friend, she felt validated that America had indeed given her a better life.

Li's hoarding had interfered with her marriage, and after her husband died, it threatened to ruin her relationship with her children. She finally realized that she had chosen stuff over her children because it was easier than working on real, honest relationships. She saw that keeping her hoarding under control was the path to a better connection with her children.

A therapist can help a hoarder explore a painful past and put that to rest. Many of the hoarders I have worked with tell me they were abused, either as children or by spouses. In therapy, Aimee was able to talk about the trauma of her abusive marriage. She started to understand that she was comforting herself by surrounding herself with things. She also realized that she was protecting herself. As a hoarder living in such extreme conditions, Aimee was subconsciously putting up a barrier that prevented anyone else from getting close to her. The hoard had become her safe haven, and living there in complete solitude felt better than risking entering another relationship, where again someone might abuse her. Aimee's therapist worked with her on trust issues, so that Aimee felt safe reaching out to people again instead of hoarding.

Hoarders with mental issues, including anxiety, depression, or OCD, need therapy as part of their treatment. Margaret refused to see a therapist to talk about what caused her anger management issues. Without treatment, I knew she was likely to slip right back into her old habits. Those deep-seated impulses don't disappear just because a house is clean. A good therapist can help hoarders understand why they do what they do, and learn to deal with their compulsions. That's when the true healing begins.

Aside from the ongoing psychological counseling, a hoarder with severe anxiety or depression may benefit from medications. Many of the hoarders I've worked with were already taking prescription drugs, and I've witnessed many cleanups go off track when a hoarder stops medication. After cleanup, I have seen hoarders feel so euphoric and confident that they quit taking their medications, thinking they don't need them. Every one of them has gone back into hoarding. When medications are involved, the addition of a therapist or medical doctor to the team is essential.

▶ Discovering Replacement Behavior

People need to feel they have a purpose in life. For a hoarder that purpose has gotten lost in the mess. When given the choice between a physical item and something as nebulous as "finding purpose," the hoarder will almost always choose the easier of the two. The goal is to help the hoarder find a suitable replacement behavior, which might be a job, volunteer work, a pastime, or a hobby—preferably one that doesn't encourage further collecting.

After Roger moved into his new, smaller house, his sister knew that he needed some form of replacement behavior, otherwise he would just sit in his house alone and almost certainly start hoarding again. Roger himself wanted some form of meaningful work, so his sister connected him with a training program for special needs workers that would try to match him with a position in which his natural obsessive-compulsive behavior might be something of an asset. Roger learned how to take warehouse inventory, and the program helped him find a job. Kathy hoped that Roger's days would be busy, and that he might even make friends.

Candace wasn't an animal hoarder, but she loved dogs. She had adopted her two Irish Setters a few years earlier, when she was working with animal rescue. Once Candace got her house cleaned up, she decided that she wanted to volunteer again with the local rescue program. She loved animals and already had experience with the program. This would allow her to spend time with dogs without endangering them. As part of the rescue program, local coordinators often made unannounced visits to the animals' foster families. Although Candace recognized that on her own she could easily get carried away and end up adopting too many dogs—and letting her house slip back into chaos—she also knew that the possibility of unannounced visits from rescue volunteers who were evaluating her home would help her keep her hoarding in check.

Volunteering forces a hoarder to think of someone else in need. The hoarder can forget momentarily about his or her own problems and feel great about helping someone or something, a meaningful connection to the rest of the world.

As a team, we try to find out a hoarder's interests. Who was this person before the hoarding started? And who does this person want to become after the cleanup? What does the hoarder enjoy: Theater? Italian food? Old movies? The conversations that members of the team can have during the cleanup support the process because we discover what is meaningful to the hoarder, and what will keep the hoarder on track after we've gone.

During cleaning, the crew essentially has a hoarder's whole life laid out in front of them and can look for clues about what hobbies the hoarder used to enjoy. Finding an old pair of hiking boots could be a starting point for conversation. Maybe the hoarder used to hike with a pet dog. Dusting off those old boots might be the first step in discovering a viable replacement therapy—and getting the hoarder out of the house and taking some valuable exercise as well.

Of course, there is always the risk that the hoarder may choose a replacement behavior that lends itself to hoarding. For example, a new hobby like cooking might trigger a hoarder to buy more pans, tools, and cookbooks than would ever be used in a lifetime.

The hoarders I've worked with who have addictive or compulsive tendencies aren't able to shut those down completely, but many have been able to channel those tendencies into more positive behaviors. Helping a hoarder choose replacement behaviors needs to be done carefully as these behaviors can be life-changing or can lead to repeating unhealthy habits.

▶ Engaging a Professional Organizer

Ongoing psychological support will help hoarders understand what they do and help them to help themselves on the road to recovery. But, just as the one-time cleanup crew will assist the hoarder in making a fresh start, sometimes it takes a professional organizer to give the hoarder the tools and advice to stay clean.

Once Nika got her house cleaned, she needed help keeping her clothing under control. She knew that she was always going to have a lot of clothes and that she would probably keep shopping. It would have been unrealistic to expect Nika to scale back too far, but making sure she organized what she had and didn't let it expand any further was an attainable goal.

Nika hired a professional organizer who set up a closet system that was tailored to Nika's specific needs—appropriate storage for her collection of shoes and purses. She also helped Nika come up with set of guidelines for deciding what to keep and what to donate, and how often to go through and evaluate her wardrobe.

While Nika only needed a few sessions with her organizer to get her closet under control, a professional can be engaged to check in with a hoarder weekly or monthly to help keep the hoarder focused—and motivated to stick with de-cluttering.

For a hoarder, staying clean isn't really about bins and labels; it's about processing items that come into the house. A good organizer can help a hoarder develop methods for sorting mail, for staying on top of recycling, and for making sure donated items get to their destinations. The organizer teaches the hoarder life skills, and the follow-up visits reinforce those skills. An organizer is like a coach, a motivator, and, occasionally, a policeman.

The repetition of bad cleaning skills is usually what got the hoarder into trouble in the first place, so an organizer works on repetition of new, positive cleaning skills. That helps the hoarder build better behaviors over the long term.

STAYING ON TRACK

While every hoarding situation may have its unique characteristics, I've found there are a number of keys that help all hoarders stay clean. Certainly, all of the elements that were discussed in the first part of this chapter are critical—self-knowledge, therapy, having a support network, focusing on more positive replacement behaviors, and so on—but the day-to-day job of staying uncluttered often requires some practical guidelines and innovative thinking. Most hoarders need guidance on a daily, sometimes hourly, basis.

Many of the ideas and exercises that follow will fall to the helpers to carry out, but most will ultimately become the responsibility of the hoarders themselves.

▶ Positive Reinforcement

Family and friends, in fact anyone on the "team" that has a continuing relationship with a hoarder, needs to understand that, like a recovering addict, a hoarder is going to struggle for the rest of his or her life. The hoarder needs to move ahead one day at a time and revel in the small successes.

When two of my workers and I showed up to take Aimee out to a celebratory lunch after her cleanup, she tried her best to look presentable. Her lipstick was all over her teeth and halfway across her face, her hair was teased into a messy pile on top of her head, and her clothes were definitely out of fashion. Did we say anything? No way. We were celebrating her big moment and enjoyed our time together with someone who only a short while earlier was leaning off the edge of her bed to use the bathroom because she was too depressed to get up and walk ten feet to the toilet.

Nika and Andre sent us photos of the Thanksgiving dinner they hosted at their house a few weeks after the cleanup. Was the dining room pristine? Of course not, but we didn't focus on the few boxes of shoes still in the corner, the worn carpet, or the peeling paint on the woodwork. We cheered them for finally inviting guests into their home.

When a hoarder first invites friends into the house, or chooses to throw away an old magazine, or tidies a two-foot-square space in the bedroom, those are all huge steps that everyone should recognize and celebrate. The goal is to build hope. There might be slipups, but positive reinforcement for even a tiny step forward encourages hoarders to realize that life can and will be better.

We leave notes around a house, in places like the bathroom mirror or inside the front door where the hoarder is sure to look every day. The notes read "You can do it!" or "You can stay clean!" This may sound corny, but hoarders tell us it makes a huge difference to be reminded that someone believes in them. The notes are a small way that we stay connected with hoarders, and they remember that we helped them clean up and that we know they can stay clean. We used to think that hoarders would eventually throw these notes out, but we have found that they keep them because they like to be reminded of how far they have come. Over time, I think the notes become small trophies throughout the home.

With hoarding, we are not just cleaning a home; we are teaching the hoarder that it is okay to love himself or herself again. We are encouraging someone who has felt worthless to feel that he or she has value and a life purpose. Positive reinforcement is about more than just giving compliments

THE SECRET LIVES OF HOARDERS

on how de-cluttered everything is. It's about noticing and reinforcing the hoarder's change in thinking and habits. It's about the hoarder moving toward new life goals and becoming a different person.

▶ Task Reminders

Posting notes around the house also serves another purpose: reminding people what needs to be done.

Like most hoarders I've worked with, Katrina responded really well to positive reinforcement. She was also able to do many jobs on her own. But because she lived alone, there was nobody to remind Katrina of her daily tasks, and also nobody to give her praise and encouragement when she followed through. To make up for this, we posted small signs all over her house. For example, she had a tendency to stack paperwork and books on the basement stairs, so we put a note on the banister that said, "Do not put papers here! Take them downstairs!" We also put up positive reinforcement cheers to bolster her clutter-free habits.

Some hoarders need reminders of daily tasks. So, for Lucy, the crafting hoarder, we added more specific guidelines: We put a note over the kitchen sink that reminded her to finish the dishes every evening and another taped to the kitchen table prompting her to take any purchased items out of their bags immediately and put them away (a common problem with shopping hoarders). Many hoarders have trouble taking out the trash or recycling, so a note on or over the trash bin can remind a hoarder that when the kitchen garbage has been bagged, to take it immediately all the way out to the outside can instead of leaving it by the back door. A note by the front door can remind a hoarder to carry the donation box out to the car as soon as it is full. And a note in the car can remind the hoarder to drop the box off at the church or other donation site.

Some hoarders I know use a "chore" chart, just like the one parents sometimes make for their kids, with gold stars for a job well done. This may sound a little juvenile, but if rewarding a fifty-five-year-old woman with gold stars (or even a big red check mark) encourages her to keep her home clean and gives her confidence and self-worth for the first time in twenty years, so be it. Hoarding is not normal; sometimes it takes unusual tools to help people.

Reminders and rewards are forever being debated in education and parenting circles, with some experts saying that parents should not reward a child for something that the child simply is supposed to do for the greater good of the family. I like that theory, but when you are dealing with a hoarder, the circumstances are quite different. For one thing, a hoarder often has had decades of repeated bad behavior, while a child is starting off fresh. Reminders and rewards should always be personalized to each hoarder's needs. We brought one hoarder her coffee each time we came to visit. If the house was clean, she got the latte; if the chores weren't done, I enjoyed a really nice coffee in front of a very sad woman. I only drank the coffee once because the chores were completed on every follow-up visit after that.

▶ Personal Space

The challenge for Jackson was that he had moved in with Mike, and both of them were concerned that Jackson's clutter might expand and take over the house they shared. Jackson was tidy; he just kept too many things. For him, the rule of "personal space" became his anti-hoarding mantra.

To establish hoarding boundaries, each family member should get a defined space in the house. For Jackson it was his closet and his own vanity and sink in the bathroom. Brad and Ellen implemented the same rule—Brad got his desk, and Ellen got the basement bookshelf. Their three children each got a large toy bin. Each family member's personal space—where it is and how big it is—needs to be agreed upon by everyone in the household. Nobody should ever "loan" personal space to another family member, because once that happens, that space is lost forever and becomes potential cause for fighting.

Everyone should agree that there won't be any arguments about what actually goes in a person's designated space (unless it's unsanitary). It doesn't matter what is being collected, just as long as it stays in its space.

The rest of the house is shared space. For anything to stay in the shared space, the family (or maybe just the adults) must agree on the item. If they can't agree, it either goes into someone's personal space, or it goes out. This rule is all about respect and boundaries.

Setting boundaries forces hoarders to live in the here and now and take responsibility for their stuff. It also prevents other household members from blaming the hoarder for all family dysfunction. Following the rules of both shared space and personal space forces the hoarder and other family members to communicate and to work together as a team to keep the home clean.

▶ A Place for Everything

Wendy had a lifetime of hoarding to overcome when Sam moved in with her. Once the house was cleaned, and their prescription drug bottle collection had been cleared out, the main problem was still that Wendy had never really learned how to organize a house. She just put things down wherever there was space, or wherever she happened to be standing. She didn't see problems with food being in the living room or dirty clothes in the kitchen.

The Ten-Minute Sweep

CANDACE TENDED TO let clutter pile up because she wasn't processing it on a daily basis. With her OCD and control issues she would put off emptying her shopping bags or clearing a table because she felt like she couldn't do it in the most perfect way possible. The main issue for Candace was to just attack clutter *daily*, before it got out of hand.

For the "ten-minute sweep," each family member (even children) chooses a specific small area to focus on. It's important to keep the cleaning area small and achievable; I suggest no more than a two-foot-square area. The person sets a timer and spends ten minutes cleaning that area. This doesn't mean just moving things from that space to a nearby chair or pile. All trash actually goes into the trash. Items to be donated need to go into the donation box. Other things that need to leave the house (library books or store returns, for example) go next to the front door, to be taken out the next day. Following through is the key. Simply shifting items from one room to another is a waste of time. Taking action and pushing through to completion is what gets an area clean.

Cleaning a house for an entire day is not realistic for most hoarders, but a ten-minute sweep is doable for even ADD hoarders who get easily distracted. The time limit gets them to micro-focus on a very specific task, and they can visually see great results immediately. Feeling good about what has been accomplished is a huge part of cleaning.

For Wendy and Sam, the best rule was "everything has a home." We made a list of their main household items and where they went—for example, pill bottles in the bathroom medicine cabinet, laundry in the hamper, and food in the kitchen cabinets. This may seem like a fundamental rule that everyone learns as a child, but many hoarders didn't pick that up either because they grew up in hoarder houses themselves, or they grew up in traumatic households where finding a meal or avoiding a beating was a daily reality. Cleaning was the least of their worries. Others may have learned but have forgotten after years of living in their own hoarder chaos.

It helps to add a guideline that like things go together. This means, for example, that clothing should be grouped: A dresser should be near the closet instead of being across the room. Bathroom supplies, like towels and extra shampoo, should be in a closet or on a shelf in or near the bathroom instead of in the kitchen pantry. A basket or drawer for incoming mail should be near the desk or table where the checkbook or computer is for paying bills. Batteries, car keys, candy, and my son's comb do not all go in the same bucket and should all go to their separate homes.

This rule works well combined with reminders posted around the home that say things like "Pill bottles don't go here—they go in the medicine cabinet." Those notes can reinforce for hoarders where things are supposed to go, especially in the early days immediately after a cleanup when the hoarder is still learning the new layout of the house.

▶ In = Out

Lucy's main issue was similar to Jackson's: She just brought far too many craft and baking supplies into the house. After her cleanup, we made the attic her "personal space" to limit her craft items. But Lucy lived alone, so there wasn't anyone there to enforce the space rule when things started to spill into other rooms of the house.

So, in addition to the "every item has a home" rule, Lucy added "in = out," meaning that whenever something new comes into the house—whether going into personal or shared space—something *of equal size* must leave. It doesn't matter if that item goes into the trash, to a donation site, or into recycling. It just needs to go out of the house immediately. For Lucy, this meant that she could only bring home a new bag of yarn if she had already used up the same amount of yarn or donated the same amount the day before. This means she would always have roughly the same volume of stuff in her house.

Hint for Shopaholics

A SHOPAHOLIC HOARDER can slip into old habits easily; the familiar excitement of finding a bargain or the overwhelming urge to buy a special gift for a loved one is strong. I recommend that such a hoarder take a buddy the first few times the hoarder shops. The friend should be prepared to ask the hoarder the tough questions: "Do you need this or just want it?" "Will it make your life better?" "Does the person for whom you are buying this really need it or just want it?" "Where will it go?" "What will you get rid of to make room for this?" This is an opportunity to help hoarders change behavior by reminding them of their rules and boundaries and concentrating on the long-term goals. (Hopefully, they have to pay cash rather than using credit cards—an even better incentive.)

IGNORING THE RULES

Sometimes hoarders just flat-out ignore their follow-up rules, either feeling like they are silly or claiming that they can stay clean without them. This is really a form of denial, and if a hoarder gets stuck here, there isn't much anyone can do. The only way a hoarder will stay clean is if the hoarder's desire to achieve an overall goal is stronger than the urge to hang on to things. It sometimes works to keep reminding the hoarder of this goal, and how the rules are the only way to reach it. I will sometimes push a little bit, saying something like "I'm not judging you about this stack of mail, but let's make sure we take care of it—right now."

If a hoarder continually refuses help, then eventually there's nothing more to do. Recovering from hoarding is a lifelong struggle, and unfortunately many people just don't make it. The reality is that not all hoarders can be saved.

At that point it is still possible to stay involved in a hoarder's life, but only if the family can stop focusing on the hoarding. The only things to do then are simply to get the hoarder out of the house frequently and work on building a relationship outside of hoarding, and continue to be positive and encouraging.

BACKSLIDING

Almost every hoarder I have worked with has had at least a few lapses back into old behaviors. I try to shut these down immediately. That means figuring out what the cause is and talking about that with the hoarder. The thing to remember is that recovery is a journey, one that the hoarder will be on for the rest of his or her life. Some backsliding is inevitable, but it doesn't mean the cleanup is a failure. It just means you have to be aware of what caused it, jump on making a change, and stay supportive.

▶ Hoarder Hangover

Many of our hoarders go through our entire mental and physical process and do everything we ask. They work hard, they let go of beloved items, they put their families first, and the home gets cleaned. They are happy that the home is cleaned, but that can turn into an elation that's just as excessive as the depression was before.

The born-again mentality is understandable because the hoarder has been paralyzed by this disease, and the cleanup and self-awareness have helped the hoarder be happy for the first time in years. Three to four days after our cleanup crew leaves, however, the reality sets in for the hoarder that all of his or her stuff is actually gone. That's when the "hoarder hangover" kicks in.

The hoarder has lost the security that he or she felt from the stuff. Often the hoarder doesn't know where anything is and freaks out. The hoarder starts to doubt the trust that was put in the cleanup crew people, and begins thinking that possessions have been stolen. The hoarder feels foolish for believing that his or her life could be gotten back together.

This is also the point at which the hoarder comes to a painful realization: The rest of his or her life troubles can no longer be blamed on the hoarding. During the hoarding phase, the hoarder has been telling himself or herself that everything else—debt, relationships, health, job—will be dealt with once the house is clean. Now the house is clean, and those problems all come crashing down on the hoarder. The hoarder hangover starts with the hoarder wanting to know where one specific item is, but within an hour it can blow up into a pounding headache of self-doubt, anger, and insecurity.

The hoarder hangover is actually good. It means the hoarder is experiencing honest emotions and is taking the process seriously. I personally believe it's a mental cleansing of all the negative feelings, just as the physical cleaning got rid of excess possessions. It's the beginning of a new phase of the hoarder's life. The hoarder phase was characterized by depression through years of living in chaos. The cleanup gave a brief high. The post-cleaning phase will hopefully be a steady rise toward a lifelong high of being clutter-free. But it will be a slow process as the hoarder deals with relinquishing bad habits, replacing behaviors, going through therapy, working with an organizer, and learning how to keep the home clean.

The hangover can last a few hours or a few days. With support and encouragement, the hoarder can usually come back to reality and keep working. I warn hoarders to expect the hangover, and tell them not to cancel any plans for the future when they are feeling anxious or low. I focus on the good that the hoarder has done.

The Emotional Roller Coaster of Hoarding

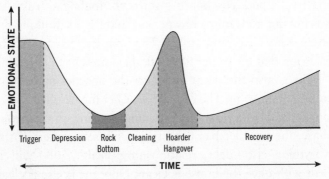

Over the years, I've had calls from clients suffering from "hoarder hangover" who are looking to understand their post-cleanup depression. I came up with this graph to show the roller coaster of hoarding. Hoarder recovery isn't a straight line—emotions will go up and down, and some stages will last longer than others. Although the hangover can be worse than the original depression, it is much easier to accept when the hoarder knows that this is a normal and often short-lived stage of the journey.

▶ Old Habits Die Hard

Even hoarders who really want to stay clean, like Nika, sometimes have trouble breaking old habits. Once her house was clean and her closets reorganized, Nika was thrilled to have so much space. But she wasn't used to it. To Nika, the de-cluttered rooms looked pretty empty compared to what she was used to. Within a few weeks, she found herself ordering some clothes from a home shopping network. She figured that a few new boxes of clothes coming in wouldn't matter because now she had room for them. She told herself it didn't mean she was starting to hoard again.

But she was hoarding again. Hoarding isn't about how much stuff someone has, it's about how they process those things. Nika's hoarding was caused by her not putting limits on herself about clothes shopping, and even though she was now only ordering a few things, her behavior could quickly escalate and clutter her house up again.

It's like a former two-pack-a-day smoker saying that he or she will only have a few cigarettes on the weekend. That looks harmless compared to the huge amounts the smoker was smoking before, but of course those few cigarettes quickly escalate until the smoker is right back to the old levels. Hoarders, like addicts, need to shut down that behavior immediately if it resurfaces. A little indulgence feels so good, and so familiar, that it will quickly grow to hoarder proportions.

For Nika, this meant following the rules, without exception. Her professional organizer had a copy of Nika's rules and was checking in with her once a week. When the organizer asked about the delivery boxes in a corner, Nika said she felt that it wasn't a big deal. The organizer reminded Nika of the "in = out" rule, and that Nika had accepted that rule during the cleanup because she wanted to reach her goal of having a better relationship with her husband. Even though a couple of boxes seemed minor, they were pointing Nika toward a path that she herself admitted she didn't want to be on again.

▶ Triggers

Whatever pushed a person to start hoarding has the potential to do it again, especially if the hoarder isn't in therapy. Aimee's divorce from an abusive man had been one of her triggers, and she did seek therapy to explore that. After a year of counseling, and carefully following the rules, Aimee was a hoarder success story. She was still clean, she had a good network of girlfriends, and she had internalized a lot of new, better habits. She was happy and involved in the outside world.

Then Aimee reconnected with an old boyfriend. At first seeing this man seemed like a positive thing for her, because it meant that she was open to relationships again. Unfortunately, this boyfriend had also been abusive, and he hadn't stopped. For Aimee, this trigger prompted her to go back into her comfort behavior.

A hoarder's family and close friends are the best ones to spot a trigger. Sometimes the event itself isn't obvious, but the sudden onset of hoarding behavior is. It's pretty likely that family members got an idea during the cleaning about what the hoarder's triggers are, and they can ask a few tactful questions to see if those are flaring up again. Ask the hoarder what he or she has been up to lately, if the hoarder has any new friends, a job change, or if the hoarder has stopped volunteering at the animal shelter.

If a trigger is the culprit, then it's time for more positive reinforcement. To a hoarder like Candace, whose OCD often held her back from completing a task, I would say something such as "I'm noticing these trash bags starting to pile up again by the back door. The last time that happened you told me it was because you weren't taking your meds. Is everything okay? Let's take these bags out while we talk about it." Hoarders are used to justifying everything, so they may assume they are being judged and get defensive. Letting hoarders know that someone cares about them, and offering to help them with the immediate task, helps them get past the defensiveness. And when hoarding behavior is triggered, even to a modest degree, it is always wise to remind hoarders of their overall goals, and how badly they want to achieve those.

Hope is a huge part of hoarding recovery. Everyone involved must believe that a hoarder can eventually be helped, or both hoarders and helpers will not have the energy to keep going when it gets tough. Most of the time it's so much easier to quit than to keep fighting. Remember that there are happy endings, and that a loving family will do anything to help. Always remember that quitting on the hoarder is yet another tragic event in the hoarder's life. Someone who wants to help a hoarder must stay focused, positive, and full of hope, because honestly, who else will?

EPILOGUE

How many of your hoarders keep their houses clean?"
Every day, people ask me about my success rate,
but the real question should be about the *hoarder* success
rate. I can help, and so can organizers, therapists, friends,
and family members, but we can only bring so much to the
table. Ultimately, whether or not a hoarder recovers is really
up to the hoarder.

Therapists I know report that 60 to 85 percent of hoarders backslide. But there have been no reliable studies to support those estimates, which don't even take into consider-
ation the fact that hoarders often make a journey through
recovery—falling off the wagon and then trying again, but
getting closer each time.

Personally, I think it's too early in the understanding of
hoarding to give a firm number, because so much depends
on the style of cleaning and the quality of follow-up counseling and guidance received. I think we will begin to
develop a deeper sense of what's possible as hoarding
becomes better understood. Right now, the best answer to
this question is that hoarders who don't follow through
with therapy and organizational support are 100 percent
guaranteed to fail.

Early- to mid-stage hoarders, Stages 1 through 3, aren't
as likely to admit they have a problem and seek help in the
first place, but once they are on board, theirs are the most

promising cases for success stories. These hoarders have fewer bad habits to break and haven't spent as much time buried in mess and becoming comfortable with it.

To stay clean, hoarders must have several of the elements of success in their favor, and early-stage hoarders are much more likely to have several of these in place. Maybe they have a terrific friend network or supportive family. Or perhaps they get heavily involved in volunteer work. Or they have a dedicated and experienced therapist. Each hoarder has different strengths and opportunities, and needs to use as many of these supports as possible. Without them, the challenge to stay clean can be overwhelming.

Stage 4 and 5 hoarders are far less likely to have classic happy endings. They may not end up the way their families hope, but if a cleanup gives them cleaner and safer lives, it's a success. Advanced hoarders have a lot more challenges on the way to what the rest of the world defines as "clean." Because of this, they need more elements of success if they are going to make it. Many of them get stuck, but even falling short of the goal is better than the life they had before.

"Success" for a hoarder is not really a goal; it's more of a journey toward a better life, even if that's not necessarily a completely clutter-free life. Some families have no hope for the hoarders in their lives. Some hoarders themselves have no hope that they can change. But everyone has the potential. Hope is what propels hoarders—and their families, friends, and helpers—through the tough process of cleaning up, and the even tougher and longer recovery period.

The stories that follow check in with several of the hoarders that we met earlier in this book. A number are out-and-out success stories by anyone's standards, and many were backsliders, but all are still on a lifetime journey of recovery.

AIMEE

Aimee, the former model and Stage 4 hoarder, could be proud of her success. After her fun lunch date with my crew to celebrate her clean house, and the lively party with her girlfriends, Aimee realized that she loved being back out in the world. She opened up like a gorgeous flower, once again sharing her sense of humor and friendly smile with everyone she met. Aimee reached out to friends and family, drawing energy and comfort from being with people instead of from hoarding.

A couple of years after her cleanup, Aimee reconnected with an old boyfriend. That Aimee was attractive and confident enough to welcome love back into her life seemed like a good sign. But then I learned that he had started to abuse her—repeating the situation with her ex-husband from which I'd thought she'd escaped. Aimee stopped returning my calls and her friends hinted that she was hoarding again.

Aimee's self-confidence was obviously still so fragile that she wasn't able to break off the damaging relationship. Instead, it triggered the familiar behavior that had helped her cope before. Aimee is a strong person, and I know she wants to have a clean house and an active, happy social life. She knows that she can stay clean if she really wants it, and I'm hopeful that she will reach the point again where she has the strength to choose that life over an abusive relationship.

MARGARET

After her cleanup, Margaret's house passed provisional inspections, but a little work still had to be done for her dogs to be returned. The inspector wanted the doors and some ceiling tiles replaced. Her plumbing and electricity were working, and the structure was sound overall. For a Stage 5 hoarder like Margaret, this was a huge success and it was probably the cleanest she would ever be.

The best part of Margaret's cleanup was when we started pulling apart the giant rat's nest we found in her mudroom, which was made up of a lot of plastic shopping bags. We opened each one, probably hundreds, and started finding cash. Apparently Margaret had a habit of shopping and tossing her change into the plastic bag. When she got home, she would pull out the microwave dinner or paper towels she had purchased, and toss the bag into the mudroom or on the kitchen floor. Who knew that rats don't eat cash? The rest of the room looked like confetti, with chewed-up paper and cardboard, but the shredded bags were guarding a small fortune: We recovered $13,000 in coins, singles, fives, and tens.

Unfortunately, the cash had to go toward the cleaning bill and paying back taxes on Margaret's property, so she didn't have much of a windfall. Her depression remained untreated because she didn't like to take her medication and she didn't cooperate with her social worker. She also didn't have much of a life outside the house. Margaret's daughter visited and their relationship improved, but Margaret still didn't have meaningful work or other connections with society. Her days looked pretty much like they had before the cleanup, except with fewer animals in the house.

Margaret still struggled to accomplish daily household tasks like washing dishes and sweeping floors. Pretty soon, trash bags were again collecting by the back door and cobwebs were taking over the corners. Margaret's daughter said that whenever she criticized Margaret for not staying on top of housework, Margaret would lose her temper and argue that it wasn't that bad. Margaret was comparing her newly clean house to how it had looked before, fully hoarded. In her mind, anything less than that was still "clean."

Unfortunately, Margaret is letting herself head right down the same path. Her house is filling up again. The good news is that it won't get as bad as it did before, because county inspectors visit about every six months, which is standard follow-up for condemned properties. If the house starts to be unsafe again, or if Margaret collects too many stray dogs, the county will serve her with another warning, and her cleanup process will begin all over again.

Margaret has family support, but not much else going for her. Most important, however, she doesn't have the true desire to change. She will probably continue to swing back and forth between hoarding and cleaning up for inspections, possibly for the rest of her life. It will definitely continue until Margaret decides that she wants something better.

BRAD AND ELLEN

After Brad and Ellen cleaned their house and put a few rules into practice, they eliminated almost all of their hoarding behavior. I'm not saying the urge isn't still there—they both realize that they have a tendency to hang on to things and to put off cleaning and de-cluttering. But they are dedicated to their rules and follow their nightly ten-minute sweep and personal space guidelines. Now the whole family is pitching in to keep the house tidy, and the kids are learning how to clean up and how to make decisions about their possessions. If a family can learn to clean together, they stay clean. If only one person does the cleaning, eventually the house gets dirty again.

Obviously what Brad and Ellen had in their favor was that they were really early-stage hoarders, so early that an outsider wouldn't even have called them hoarders. They didn't have a lot of clutter in the house, but they were developing hoarder mind-sets. Either one of them could easily slip more deeply into hoarding, but because they were able to change their thinking early on, it's probably not going to be an issue for them moving forward.

LI

Li's cleanup of her large house and barn went really smoothly because her children had laid the groundwork in advance. The family had already agreed on the few items they wanted to uncover and keep, and Li said that the rest could go, which meant Li wasn't agonizing over every little thing. With her daughter, Sunny, overseeing the work and calling Li whenever we found something on her "fire list," the crew whisked through the house and barn in a few days.

At first, Li was delighted with her newly empty house. But after making a few minor repairs during the following months, she started feeling a little lost and alone in her big house, even though her children and grandchildren were visiting. Eventually, she decided to put the place on the market and move into an assisted living facility nearby.

Li moved into her new apartment and jumped right into activities and making friends. I've seen many hoarders go to assisted living and hide in their rooms and continue to hoard, but Li busied herself playing bridge, mah-jongg, and going to lunch with friends. Once Li filled her life with people and events, she found that she didn't have time or a need for hoarding anymore. Li is exceptional, if not unique, for a late-stage hoarder. Today, Li is living happily in her apartment, clutter-free. And she still looks fabulous.

RICK

Even with his advancing dementia, Rick had a successful cleanup aided by his sister. An early-stage hoarder, Rick was willing to let his house go, which motivated him to clean it up for the sale. Although he was sometimes confused during the cleanup, by the end he had only about a dozen boxes to go into storage in his sister's basement.

Rick didn't have many outside interests. As a retired professor, he occasionally attended university events, but his sister realized that even these outings would start to taper off as his dementia worsened. Given his mental status, it would have been highly likely that Rick would revert to his hoarding habits except that he was able to live with his sister. She not only kept a clean house but also encouraged him to maintain a social life of sorts by staying in touch with other retired professors and friends from his university community.

JACKSON

I wish I could say that every hoarder turns out like Jackson. Jackson definitely had a few struggles after we cleaned his house, and he will probably have a few more in his future, but he ultimately had a happy ending. After working with Jackson for most of a week, we left him to de-clutter the rest of his house on his own. His partner, Mike, reported that Jackson made progress for the first few months. But six months after the cleaning, we got a call from Mike saying that Jackson had stalled. He wasn't bringing new items into the house, which was terrific news. But he'd had a setback when someone broke into the house. While nothing valuable was taken, it took Jackson a few weeks to process the event.

Much to everyone's relief, Jackson took the violation as a challenge. He decided to use it to push through, finish the job, and redefine himself as someone who was no longer a hoarder. That doesn't mean he wasn't tempted to withdraw into his comfort behavior. But Jackson had Mike to talk through that with him and offer support and understanding. It was hard and emotionally risky for Jackson, but he chose the right path instead.

Mike called me later to report that Jackson had finally finished cleaning out the house on his own and put it on the market. He kept some of his most important Blondie collectibles to display, including signed record album covers. As an early-stage hoarder with lots of support, he was able to weather many of the challenges that he faced. Today, the two of them are living happily together in Mike's house, complete with Cher's doorknobs, and Jackson is learning to control his hoarding tendencies.

KATRINA

Katrina got most of her Stage 3 house clean in four days working alongside us and was seeing her therapist for depression. The house looked a little like what it must have when she first moved in, a decade earlier, with its streamlined white kitchen, pale carpets, and modern living room.

Katrina hoped that her daughter and son-in-law would bring their two girls for a weekend visit soon, but they wanted her to finish the two remaining bedrooms that were still cluttered with all of her legal documents, relating to her law school education and her divorce, and the boxes of her skin care products and catalogs.

Katrina wanted to get those rooms done, but she struggled. For a month after the cleaning, one of our crew went to help Katrina for a few hours one day a week. When they worked together, she was able to get through a few boxes, but that didn't make much headway into the two full rooms. After our visits stopped, Katrina slipped more deeply into her depression. She stopped seeing her therapist, and she gave up on finishing the de-cluttering.

Without therapy, Katrina lost a critical pillar of support. And although her daughter was loving and offered encouragement to finish the cleanup, she lived too far away to give her mother the kind of regular support she needed. Katrina didn't have much involvement in outside activities, and most of her friends had drifted away when her hoarding increased.

Despite all those strikes against her, Katrina managed to keep her house clean. In her favor, she still had a fulfilling job and a very supportive boss who gave her time off to do her cleanup. Six months after we worked with her, she still had full use of her kitchen, living room, bathroom, and bedroom. Katrina wasn't bringing new stuff into the house, not even into the two full "storage" rooms.

Katrina had made tremendous progress and she was finally living in a clean, safe environment. I'm confident that Katrina can maintain the status quo. She will probably need help emptying those two bedrooms, and she may call us within a year or so and say that she's ready to get that done. First, she will have to deal with her depression and develop some outside friendships.

In the meantime, when I talk to Katrina I give her lots of praise for keeping the rest of her house clean, and remind her of what huge improvements she has already made in her life. She's moving forward in the journey to stay clean.

MARCIE

Cleaning Marcie's house started off pretty well. The living room was filled up to the ceiling with piles of stuff Marcie had bought—much of which had never been taken out of its original packaging. The room was so full that it took my crew about two days just to get through that one room. Once Marcie let us into her house and accepted that we were there to help her, she was right with us on that first day, making decisions on what stayed, what was to be donated, and what was trash. She was making good progress.

On the second day Marcie and I had the talk about her abusive husband. She admitted that she shopped to comfort herself, and I'm guessing that he gave her money because he felt guilty.

When the realization about why she hoarded hit her, Marcie ran through her pathways to the kitchen where her husband was. I could hear her shouting, "I do this because you hit me!" He was built like a linebacker, over six and a half feet tall with solid shoulders. Although he was eighty, he wasn't frail or stooped. When he came out of the back of the house and took a swing at me, I knew I didn't want to get into a fistfight with him. We left, planning to come back the next day after the drama had calmed down.

This was clearly a case where a psychologist could have helped, but unfortunately Marcie didn't have that support, which as a late-stage hoarder she could really have used. As the crew and I were having breakfast in the hotel restaurant, I was served with a restraining order, and we were never allowed back. It's one of the few hoarder houses that I started but didn't finish. We have stayed in touch with Marcie's children, but she still lives with her husband in that home of clutter and abuse, and she will probably stay there for the rest of her life unless she makes the decision to leave.

Abuse, like hoarding, is something that will continue until the person at risk decides to make a change. Unfortunately, even if a hoarder is in a dangerous situation, like Marcie, not much can be done if she chooses to stay there. In her case, the hoarding is really the least of her worries. At the moment, Marcie just has too many other critical issues going on to deal with her hoarding.

LUCY

Lucy's relationship with her family was strained and complicated. Ever since her daughter spearheaded a secret cleanup a few years before I was called in, Lucy had been hanging on to anger and resentment over the disrespectful way she felt treated. But when her house filled up again and got to the point where Lucy couldn't stay there, her daughter reached out and invited Lucy to stay with her.

We classified Lucy as a mid-stage hoarder who still had many issues to work through. Even during and after her cleanup, Lucy continued to live with her daughter, and as her collection of craft supplies dwindled at her own house, Lucy tried to carry some yarn and fabric to her daughter's house to keep. The daughter drew a line and told Lucy that wasn't acceptable.

Lucy's daughter also encouraged her to move back into her own house once it was in livable condition. While Lucy might have seen this suggestion as a rejection, her children softened the blow by spending time with Lucy doing fun things outside the house.

Lucy moved back into her own house and began to see a therapist. It seemed like she had a lot going for her, with supportive children and professional counseling, but only a month after hear cleanup, Lucy went back to hoarding.

In the first few weeks after her cleanup, my crew or I checked on Lucy weekly. When I'd called to tell her I was coming by the next day, I discovered, she would stay up all night cleaning out her living room and moving things to the attic. She became a sort of *bulimic hoarder*, falling into a cycle of hoarding and then purging.

One problem for Lucy was that her therapist didn't seem to get any insight into the extent of her issues. The therapist had never seen her house or spoken with her children. Like many hoarders, Lucy was saying the right things to hide her problem. She said that the therapist told her that she was doing just fine.

Aside from the lack of help she got from therapy, Lucy had also lost her main connection with the world when she retired, which contributed to a somewhat bleak picture of her situation. She was hoarding again, and she didn't appear to have much incentive to stop. But for now, I still have to give Lucy a thumbs-up. The fact is that her relationship with her kids got much better after the cleanup. They used to yell at one another about the hoarding, but afterward they started to focus less on the hoarding and more on enjoying one another's company outside the house.

Lucy is still trying, and her life got better, just not quite to where her family hoped it could be. Sometimes the family wants a cleanup much more than the hoarder does. That's when the family just has to accept the relationship for what it is.

NIKA

Nika started off well, meeting with her organizer once a week. But after she started buying clothes again a few months after her cleanup, she canceled her organizer appointment. The organizer called Nika a few more times, but she never heard back. Eventually she gave up.

Even though she was a mid-stage hoarder, I was concerned about Nika because during her cleaning I noticed that her husband, Andre, understandably, wasn't very encouraging. He had lived with this for years and had doubts. He was eager for the house to be clean, but he had adopted an attitude of "I'll believe it when I see it." Living with someone who was skeptical instead of supportive made it easy for Nika to let herself off the hook. If Andre didn't think it was possible, why would Nika even bother to try? The lack of support was Nika's main challenge.

I suspect that Nika decided that the organizer was pushing her too hard, and she just gave up on trying. Mid-stage hoarders like Nika have a good chance for a full recovery, but only if they have a few key factors in their favor. Support from loved ones can help these hoarders gather the energy to fight years of bad habits. Or therapy and organizational tips can give highly motivated hoarders the tools they need to build new habits and ways of thinking. Nika had a great organizer, but not the motivation or support to stick with it.

Once she quit meeting with her organizer, Nika didn't have any elements of success working in her favor. I haven't heard from her since her cleanup, and although her house is no doubt cleaner and she is in a better situation than before, I suspect she is still buying clothes.

ROXANNE

Roxanne had been hoarding in her trailer home ever since her children were young. She was forced to clean up at age sixty at her social worker's insistence, so that home health care could safely visit the house.

At her age and given the amount of time she had been hoarding, it would have been a struggle for anyone to change those entrenched habits. Even though we might think of her as only a mid-stage hoarder, Roxanne had the additional challenge of being poor. A lifelong smoker and heavy drinker, she had developed throat cancer. Her liver was failing and she had to wear a colostomy bag. Doctors had told Roxanne that even with treatment, her time was short. Her goal was to get the trailer de-cluttered enough for hospice to be able to care for her during the cancer's end stages, and we did that.

Roxanne had no family support. Her daughter hadn't visited in ten years, and although the social worker had contacted her and explained Roxanne's situation, the daughter wasn't interested. Roxanne also didn't have any friends, and her neighbors in the trailer park had been avoiding her for years.

Roxanne had no loved ones supporting her, no motivation to change, and limited time and physical energy. She had decades of hoarding under her belt and she was stuck in a fantasy past. She had resisted therapy and she had no outside interests. Roxanne had too many strikes against her for an effective recovery.

A few months later, we got news from the social worker that Roxanne's cancer had gone into remission and she no longer needed hospice care.

That was a remarkable gift for Roxanne, but unfortunately, without other positive support in her life, I can only imagine that if she is still with us, Roxanne's sitting in that smoke-filled trailer, full of stuff, waiting for her daughter to visit.

BEN

I stop by to visit Ben, the "pizza man" and late-stage hoarder, every few months to encourage him to let me help clean out his house, but he's still not interested. Now he has three identical Volvo station wagons, each filled to the brim with empty pizza boxes, half-used bottles of pizza sauce, old pepperoni, and other food trash. At this point, the three cars have cost him more than it would have cost to clean up the house. Ben will probably have to buy a fourth car pretty soon and start filling that up. The house is definitely a Stage 5 situation, and his neighbors are starting to complain because the airplane and car parts are spilling out into the yard.

Ben is still in denial about his hoarding. When I mention it, he will talk about it for a few minutes but then change the subject. He can talk your ear off about almost any topic, but

Ben won't talk about his hoarding, or the fact that his wife and kids have left him because of it. I keep reminding him that I care enough to help him get his life back, but I expect that Ben won't do anything until he is forced to. Eventually a building inspector will visit, and the process of condemning Ben's property will begin.

The only way a cleanup can help Ben is if he admits that he has a problem that is ruining his life, and decides he wants to change it. Unless he can do that, Ben will end up just like Margaret, waffling between clean and cluttered for the rest of his life, and resenting "those people" who keep making him get rid of his valuable stuff. It's really a shame. The man is brilliant and could add so much to so many lives. Instead he chooses to live a lie in complete solitude with his stuff when he could be acknowledging the truth and working toward recovery.

CANDACE

With her OCD, alcoholism, grief over her mother's death, and advanced Stage 4 house, Candace seemed like a hoarder who had an overwhelming number of barriers to staying clean. Any one of those issues could keep her stuck in hoarding, but Candace is a strong woman who brought real enthusiasm to her recovery. However, she got bogged down in several challenges.

Before we would even take her cleanup job, I told Candace that she had to stop drinking. She poured out her liquor and started attending AA meetings again. She threw herself into the cleaning. Afterward, she started getting estimates for repairs and for adapting one of her spare rooms for temporarily fostering rescue dogs.

Candace was on a high after her cleanup; she was thrilled to have her life back. She was full of energy and plans for a promising new future. But a few weeks later, Candace slipped into the hoarder hangover. Because Candace didn't have much of a life outside her hoarding, she got stuck feeling unsure of who her new "self" was. Candace felt overwhelmed by the repairs she had planned. It felt to her like she had taken on too much too soon, and she slipped back into some of her former comfort behavior. She stopped seeing her therapist and quit taking her OCD medication. Then she started drinking again.

Candace had a lot of challenges and not very many support tools. She didn't have family or close friends, only her AA meeting contacts. She tried attending a hoarder support group, but she felt that was depressing instead of encouraging.

In addition, Candace discovered that she was $10,000 more in debt than she'd originally calculated, as a result of credit card abuse. As her hoarding got worse, she had started losing or throwing away her credit card bills. Now she couldn't afford to make the repairs to her house, and without those repairs, her plans to volunteer with the ASPCA were on hold.

Even with those challenges, the good news is that Candace's house hasn't gotten any worse. Her life is better than it was two years ago, and she is trying to reach out and connect with people again. For Candace, like most late-stage hoarders, it's very tempting to give up instead of doing the hard work to get her life back together. Candace may be taking a little break, but I'm proud of her for making it this far and I'm hopeful that she has the energy to keep moving toward her goals. Candace's story is not finished, and only she can decide if she'll continue to live in depression and mess or if she'll take all the necessary steps and get the help she needs.

THALIA

After locking herself in her car and threatening to swallow a bottle of pills, Thalia was taken to the hospital immediately. The cleanup was put on hold because obviously we couldn't make any decisions about what to keep or throw away without guidance from her. Cleaning while she was gone would have made the situation worse.

Fortunately, Thalia's attempted suicide was more a cry for help than an actual attempt, and one to which members of her support network were able to respond. Her therapist made sure that Thalia got treatment, and when she returned to the house, we finished her cleanup.

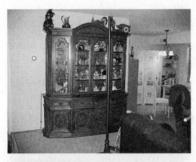

At the end of Thalia's cleanup things were looking good.

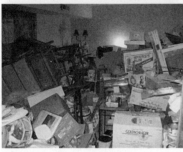

Two years after Thalia's cleanup she'd reverted to her old habits—and then some. It's our policy not to do a second cleanup except under really exceptional circumstances. We weren't able to help Thalia until she was ready to help herself.

But Thalia was a classic late-stage hoarder and still in denial. She cleaned up in order to keep her house, not because she wanted to give up hoarding. Two years later Thalia called and confessed that her house was full again. But as we talked, it became clear that she was still in denial and only wanted to clean up enough so that her house wouldn't be condemned a second time. I knew that if we came and cleaned, the same cycle would repeat itself, and so I turned her down. I told her that if she gets to the point where she really wants to change, I'll be her biggest supporter.

ROGER

We are all still rooting hard for Roger. During his cleanup, he started out by not trusting the crew at all. He didn't have faith in anyone apart from his sister Kathy. But partway through the job, he opened up and bonded with the group. Once he realized that we weren't going to lie to him or throw away his stuff without his permission, he became much more communicative and friendly. He would talk sports all day long; he had a brilliant mind for details and statistics. The happiest I saw him was when he earned a Clutter Cleaner shirt on day two of his cleanup. This kind of thing, in itself, is a great victory for an advanced hoarder.

As Roger shared stories with us, and his sister did also, we learned that Roger had several serious challenges. He had been abused as a child by someone he trusted outside of the family, and that had scarred him emotionally. His parents had let Roger live with them so that they could, in a way, protect him from his fears and the outside world. When they died, Roger felt almost completely alone. Therapy wasn't an option—not only was the closest therapist two hours away, but Roger didn't trust anyone enough to even try counseling.

The cleaning led to Roger suffering another big loss—the sale of the family house. He moved to a smaller house nearby. With so many of his things having been thrown away in the cleanup, he struggled emotionally. His sister Kathy was patient and supportive, and would have done almost anything for him. She helped him land a job, and for a while it looked like Roger was on a good path toward recovery.

The job doing inventory in a warehouse had been located through an organization that trained and found placement for workers with special needs. But Roger had been living alone and on his own terms for so long that he wasn't able to meet some basic societal expectations. He couldn't get to work on time. And when he did show up, he had not bathed, had food stains on his clothes, and crunchy things in his beard. He had trouble staying focused and carrying on simple conversations.

Roger was let go. After that, he went back to hoarding.

Roger's family had done everything right, and Roger worked hard. But without therapy and some connection to the outside world, he couldn't maintain a clutter-free house. Kathy isn't sure that Roger can ever live alone, and he may need home health care support to make sure he eats and bathes.

Roger's family is dedicated to supporting him and making sure he has a place to live, but at this point, Kathy feels like she has tried everything to help him be clean. She is working on accepting and loving Roger for who he is.

Advanced hoarders are all on the same journey that Roger is, moving back and forth along a continuum from clutter to tidy. Their goal may be merely to stay closer to the clean end of the scale, and their loved ones need to be content with that. Luckily, Roger's living conditions are safe, and his family is accepting the reality of his situation.

WENDY AND SAM

After their cleanup and meetings with social workers and doctors to talk about the prescription pill hoarding, newly-wed seniors Wendy and Sam were able to keep their house clean by following some rules and checklists. Sam, who had never been a hoarder, wasn't really contributing to the problem, and he was able to support Wendy, an early-stage hoarder herself, in her efforts to stay clean. Because she wanted this new relationship to work, Wendy had the motivation to stick with it.

Wendy's adult daughter and young granddaughter had been living with them, but after the cleanup Wendy realized that having extra people in the house was a stress button for her. Also, her daughter, having grown up in a hoarder house, had hoarding tendencies herself. She and the granddaughter were working on turning that around by applying the same cleanup rules Wendy and Sam had. But Wendy could see that it was a struggle to have four people in a small house, with at least two of them being recovering hoarders. She asked her daughter to find her own apartment.

Once the house was clean, Wendy and Sam were faced with maintenance issues that Wendy had ignored for years. Also, for the first time ever, they were doing weekly cleaning—dusting, vacuuming, and washing dishes. They decided that the house was just too much work for them to maintain. After Wendy's daughter moved out, Wendy and Sam put the house on the market with the goal of moving to a smaller low-maintenance space.

Throughout the process, Wendy was being honest with herself, and by moving, she imposed space limits on herself. With this, combined with her newly learned cleaning techniques and the support from her children, hers has become a success story.

MICHELLE

Once her house was clean and de-moused, Michelle's two children were returned to her from foster care. Michelle responded well to antianxiety medication. The house stayed clean, so Michelle's social worker considered her a success story. As far as he could see, Michelle had cleaned up, passed inspection, gotten her children back, and was in compliance with her medications. So he closed her case.

A few months after, Michelle decided that she felt so great and things were going so well that she didn't need her medication anymore. Once she quit taking it, she slipped back into anxiety and hoarding, not an unlikely scenario for a Stage 5 hoarder. The house isn't as bad as it was before, but Michelle is definitely on that same path again.

During Michelle's cleaning we had found some drugs in the house, which she said her son had brought in. About a year after the cleanup, I heard from Michelle's case worker that Michelle's son had been convicted on a separate drug-related charge and was serving time in jail.

Her daughter is still in the house, but she is a teenager and will be moving out soon. After that, unfortunately, there won't be much incentive for Michelle to stay clean. She could easily continue to hoard and fill up the house until neighbors start to complain and city inspectors visit again.

DAISY

Miss Daisy had a remarkable recovery for an elderly Stage 5 hoarder. She had several positive factors working for her. One was her terrific support team. Another was the fact that she hadn't been a hoarder all of her life. Daisy didn't start hoarding until after her retirement, so she had experienced what a tidy house felt like, and she understood how to keep it that way. She appreciated order and knew that she had the tools to reach that goal and stay there.

Even though Daisy was in her eighties, she had an alert mind and good health. And her cleaning turned up a string

THE SECRET LIVES OF HOARDERS

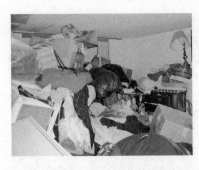

With Daisy's clutter piled almost to the ceiling, the cleanup crew was afraid of what they might find under it all.

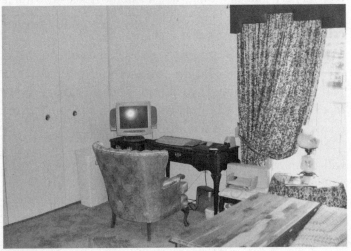

Daisy had a remarkable team of helpers who got her bedroom livable again.

of positives that helped encourage her. First, when her county-provided financial planner learned that Daisy had been a teacher for thirty years, he did a little research and discovered an $85,000 pension that Daisy didn't know she had. Using that, he put together a budget that ensured Daisy would be taken care of for the rest of her life. That was a huge positive that proved to Daisy the benefits of cleaning up and organizing her life.

Meanwhile, Daisy's social worker located family members who were living nearby. Daisy had cut off contact with them fifteen years earlier, embarrassed by her hoarding.

They thought Daisy had passed away and were thrilled to find her alive and well. Her family welcomed Daisy back into their lives unconditionally, delighted to have their mother, grandmother, and great-grandmother back.

Daisy also had her strong church community. She had volunteered there for years and had endless support and love from the large congregation. That gave her life meaning. Each day when Daisy got up, she had somewhere to go and people who needed her.

With her pension, Daisy could have lived on her own after her house was cleaned. Instead, her family kept asking her to move in with them. She finally decided to sell her house and live with one of her adult grandchildren. She is still there today, in her nineties, volunteering at her church and spending time with her great-grandchildren.

RESOURCES

By the planning stage, people usually have hundreds of questions about where to get special tools, or where to donate some items, or simply who to call for more help. As the understanding of hoarding grows, additional resources will become available and added to the resource list on our website at www.cluttercleaner.com.

Most of the resources listed here have national coverage, but always look for local solutions as well (key words to search for are included under each topic). Local companies may be able to help find nearby support for other aspects of the project.

ABOUT HOARDING

The resource section that follows features additional information about the basics of hoarding, including therapists, cleaning companies, and support groups available. To find more information, keywords to search include hoarding, squalor, OCD, saving, collecting, clutter, and organization.

Institute for Challenging Disorganization (ICD):
www.challengingdisorganization.org
International Obsessive-Compulsive Disorder (OCD)
Foundation: www.ocfoundation.org

National Association of Professional Organizers
(NAPO): www.napo.net
A&E's *Hoarders*: www.aetv.com/hoarders

TREATMENT CENTERS

Hoarding can have multiple triggers and accompanying mental health–related issues. Following are some of the top treatment centers in the country for hoarding, anxiety, OCD, and related disorders. Most cities and many universities also have local specialists. To find more information, keywords include OCD, obsessive-compulsive disorder, hoarding, phobia, anxiety, depression, stress, body dysmorphic disorder, trichotillomania, panic, agoraphobia, social anxiety, and PTSD.

Lakeside Center for Behavioral Change (Dr. Renae Reinardy): www.lakesidecenter.org
Kansas City Center for Anxiety Treatment (Dr. Lisa Hale): www.kcanxiety.com
The Institute of Living (Dr. David Tolin): www.compulsivehoarding.org
Panic/Anxiety/Recovery Center (PARC): www.beyondanxiety.com
Compulsive Hoarding Center (Dr. Robin Zasio): www.compulsivehoardingcenter.com
Obsessive-Compulsive Disorder Institute of Greater New Orleans (Dr. Suzanne Chabaud): www.ocdigno.com

SUPPORT GROUPS

Most localities do not have physical support groups for family members of hoarders or for hoarders themselves, but that is changing. Meanwhile, there are multiple support groups online. These grow and change quickly, so to stay current on what's available, search on the following keywords: hoarding support, squalor support, organizational therapy, families of hoarding, and children of hoarding.

Children of Hoarders: www.childrenofhoarders.com
(This site also features a valuable resource page of general hoarding information.)
Clutterers Anonymous: www.clutterersanonymous.net
Squalor Survivors: www.squalorsurvivors.com
Mates of Messies: http://groups.yahoo.com/group/
Mates-of-Messies/

ANIMAL HOARDING

Animal hoarding is a growing disorder that is receiving increasing attention, with more and more resources and research becoming available. Please be aware that the pictures on some of these websites are graphic and can be disturbing. Additional information can be found by searching for these keywords: animal hoarding, animal abuse, pet abuse, animal cruelty, and foreclosure pets.

ASPCA: www.aspca.org
Humane Society: www.humanesociety.org
Pet Abuse: www.pet-abuse.com/pages/animal_cruelty/
hoarding.php

Animal Legal Defense Fund: www.aldf.org
Hoarding of Animals Research Consortium:
www.tufts.edu/vet/hoarding/harc.htm

GENERAL PSYCHOLOGY

For a hoarding cleanup to be successful, it is important for hoarders to get a better understanding of what is the trigger and why they hoard. I encourage all hoarders and family or friends affected by hoarding to seek therapy if needed. Below is a list of websites that can lead to local therapists who can help with long-term treatment. Keywords include psychology, therapy, cognitive therapy, social workers, abuse, divorce, grief, and separation.

Association for Behavioral and Cognitive Therapies:
www.abct.org (searchable national therapist list)
Awareness Foundation for OCD and Related Disorders: www.ocdawareness.com
American Psychological Association: www.apa.org
Anxiety Disorders Association of America:
www.adaa.org (searchable national therapist list)

BOOKS

We have written an overview of hoarding—what it is, why it happens, and how to help. These books are helpful to learn more specifics about the disorder and how to work with it, for understanding the psychology of hoarding, and for step-by-step suggestions on how to organize a house so that it stays clean.

THE SECRET LIVES OF HOARDERS

Digging Out: Helping Your Loved One Manage Clutter, Hoarding, and Compulsive Acquiring by Michael A. Tompkins and Tamara L. Hartl (New Harbinger Publications, 2009)

Stuff: Compulsive Hoarding and the Meaning of Things by Randy O. Frost and Gail Steketee (Houghton Mifflin, 2010)

Buried in Treasures: Help for Compulsive Acquiring, Saving, and Hoarding by David F. Tolin, Randy O. Frost, and Gail Steketee (Oxford University Press, 2007)

Overcoming Compulsive Hoarding by Fugen Neziroglu, Jerome Bubrick, and Jose Yaryura-Tobias (New Harbinger Publications, 2004)

It's All Too Much: An Easy Plan for Living a Richer Life with Less Stuff by Peter Walsh (Free Press, 2007)

CLEANING

Some families may try to clean the home themselves and some families may bring in a professional. Regardless of how the home gets cleaned, it's important to explore all options before making a final decision. Remember that it sometimes takes a hoarder decades to clutter up a house, and it won't take one weekend to get it empty. Safety and price are the key factors to consider when deciding on a physical cleaning process.

Cleaning Services

There are very few professional cleaning companies in the United States that can handle both the mental and physical requirements of a hoarding cleanup, although that will likely change. Before hiring someone to clean a home, please research the company thoroughly, ask for references and proof of insurance, and find out how many hoarders the company has worked with. Ask about success rates and ask to speak with hoarder clients, not just the family member who hired the company. The company 1-800-GOT-JUNK can handle Stage 1 or 2 hoarding, when the job focuses just on debris removal and not mental issues. The other two companies can take any job up to a Stage 5.

Clutter Cleaner: www.cluttercleaner.com
SteriClean: www.steri-clean.com
1-800-GOT-JUNK: www.1800gotjunk.com

ORGANIZERS

Some organizers can clean a Stage 3 house and higher, but most are better for aftercare than the initial cleanup. The organizer can teach ongoing skills to the hoarder. As with the cleaning services, research the options and get to know the organizer before hiring. This person will be working side by side with the hoarder, so make sure their personalities match. Look for Certified Professional Organizer (CPO) certification for more extreme cases.

National Association of Professional Organizers (with a searchable directory): www.napo.net
Metropolitan Organizing, LLC (Geralin Thomas): www.metropolitanorganizing.com
Abundance Organizing: www.abundanceorganizing.com
The Delphi Center for Organization (Dorothy Breininger): www.delphicenterfororganization.com

Things in Place (Standolyn Robertson):
    www.thingsinplace.com
Dr. DClutter Life Management: (Dr. Darnita Payden):
    www.drdclutter.com

SUPPLIES

Every job will need lots of different supplies, most of which can be picked up at any local or national hardware or home improvement store. The most important items are listed below.

Clothing

- Steel-toe boots
- Long socks and pants
- Long-sleeve shirts
- Tyvec protective suits with hood (when needed)
- Work gloves with latex coating to keep liquids from seeping in (Use tight-fitting gloves and avoid big, bulky leather gloves that won't give much flexibility.)
- Respirators or masks (Make sure they read P100 or N95. If it doesn't say either on the mask, do not wear it into the house.)

Cleaning Supplies

- 3-millimeter-thick trash bags
- Cardboard boxes for sorting only, not to be used for storing items
- Labels and permanent markers
- Pocketknife or box cutter to open old boxes and cut strings

- All-purpose cleaner
- Paper towels
- Brooms, snow shovels, and rakes

OTHER SERVICES

Dumpsters

If the family is not hiring a professional junk removal company to help, a Dumpster is indispensable. Try to find a thirty-cubic-yard Dumpster or larger (a cubic yard is roughly the equivalent size of a dishwasher). Some cities will require a permit if the Dumpster is stored on the street. If at all possible, have the Dumpster full each night so it can be picked up early the next morning.

Waste Management: www.wm.com

Document Shredding

Most houses need document shredding because of old tax and financial papers, medical records, and other secure information. I recommend calling a document shredding company that will come to the hoarder's house, shred on-site, and give the hoarder a certificate showing that the documents have been shredded.

Shred It: www.shredit.com

Portable Storage

If storage is necessary, we recommend portable storage, which can be easily dropped off and picked up at any time. We tend to work with SmartBox USA because their boxes are the perfect size for sorting, shipping, and storage. They charge a monthly fee.

Smartbox USA: www.smartboxusa.com

Pest Control

I recommend having a contact number handy in case spiders, rats, mice, fire ants, or roaches appear during cleaning. The hoarder may already be aware of what infestations are in the house. Look online for a local provider. Keywords are pest, rodent control, critter, and the name of any specific insect or animal in the house.

Prescription Drug Disposal

One way for clearing out used or expired prescription medication is to call a local veterinarian's office or police department, as both process large amounts of controlled substances. Also check with local pharmacies, as many of them have national bag campaigns in which customers can fill a bag and the pharmacy will mail it to the FDA to be destroyed (free of charge).

EPA

It's possible that the house may have some chemicals that are no longer safe. Have a list of the chemicals and call the EPA one time to discuss disposal options. They will most likely point the resident in the direction of a local dump on a special day, but it never hurts to contact the EPA first. Many professional cleaning companies will take care of this for the family.

Environmental Protection Agency: www.epa.gov

Bio-waste

If the house has alarming amounts of feces, urine, or medical waste, then the family should most likely hire a professional service. But if the family has questions during the research phase, I suggest contacting the company below and asking about their medical waste pickup.

Stericycle: www.stericycle.com

REMOVAL

We've found that many hoarders are in financially challenging situations and could use a few extra dollars. Although few sales of hoarded items yield financial windfalls, these resources are the best opportunity to earn some cash or a tax deduction.

Donation

Salvation Army: www.salvationarmyusa.org
Goodwill: www.goodwill.org
Craigslist: www.craigslist.org
Freecycle: www.freecycle.org

Appraisers and Auction Houses

Having a yard sale or estate sale is rarely worth the effort. We only work with auction houses, which typically take between 25 and 35 percent of the sale to cover their expenses.

American Society of Appraisers (Find an Appraiser tool): www.appraisers.com

Antiques Roadshow (listing of appraisers by name or
   specialty): www.pbs.org/wgbh/roadshow/appraisers
   /index.html
International Society of Appraisers (searchable mem-
   bership database): www.isa-appraisers.org
Auction Guide: www.auctionguide.com
National Auctioneers Association: www.auctioneers.org

Home Shopping Networks

Most home shopping networks will accept recent returns on
merchandise still in the packaging (obviously it must be
clean). Call to ask about the options, and if the first customer service representative says no, then speak with a manager and explain the situation.

Scrap Metal

Scrap metal prices fluctuate according to the economy and
time of year. Local scrap metal yards can quote prices for
"separated" and "mixed" scrap. Unless the aluminum and
copper are already separated, they will pay the lower
"mixed" rate. Get a receipt and make sure the rate per ton
matches the quote over the phone.

   If delivering the metal isn't an option, ask the local scrap
yard if they can recommend a delivery service (expect to
split the proceeds fifty-fifty with that service). For junked
cars, most localities will insist that the registration and title
are present before scrapping the car.

THE SECRET LIVES OF HOARDERS

ACKNOWLEDGMENTS

I've always believed that opportunities can show themselves at any time. The first time I met my writing partner, Phaedra Hise, I learned that the magazine she worked for had just folded. I ended up paying for the coffee, but by that afternoon I had a literary agent and a rough draft for a book proposal. I must thank Phaedra for working side by side with me on this project and crafting my ramblings into purposeful stories with action and direction. Phaedra turned her life upside down to make this book happen, and I could never thank her enough. I also want to thank Jane Dystel at Dystel & Goderich Literary Management for putting her name behind mine and having the guts to discuss hoarding before it was cool. Most important, thanks to my publisher, John Duff, for having the vision to see that a trash guy with a blackjack problem could help millions of people understand hoarding. *The Secret Lives of Hoarders* would not exist if John had not put his money and his mouth behind this project. I greatly appreciate his guidance, support, and wisdom.

I first understood the idea of opportunities showing themselves at any time after my father died, which prompted me to get involved in a bereavement camp for children called Comfort Zone Camp in Richmond, Virginia. Volunteering at this camp helped me not only to learn how to deal with grief—and help others do so—but to understand myself better and to literally find myself. I now have a business, a wife, and a son because of my time there. During his lifetime, my father taught me to work passionately and keep a wicked sense of humor. A big thank-you to Ed Paxton, who is missed every day.

Thanks especially to A&E Television Networks and specifically Andy Berg for giving me the opportunity to be on television and to help hoarders. Thanks to the entire staff at Screaming Flea Productions Inc. and the crew for encouraging me to be myself and for making *Hoarders* an incredible show. A special thanks to the amazing Dr. Suzanne Chabaud for adding to this book and for being an awesome travel companion. Thanks also to the Caplan family and to the Harrington family (especially Sean for letting me stay in his house while I figured out my entire life). And thank you to my Australian friends, Marcus and Thomas: I only understand half of what they say, but even half is enough to make a difference in my life.

I truly appreciate the support of my friends and family on this journey. I owe my uncle John for driving across the country on my first business adventure and teaching me the joy of figuring it out along the way. The women in my life pushed me to be the man I am today, and I love them all: Nanny, Be-Be, Jane, and Spiker. Be-Be taught me much more than she will ever know, and I appreciate the wonderfully eccentric lady that she is. My mom always believed in me even though she just wanted me to get a real job. I know that she is proud and that's all I ever wanted. This book was born around the same time as my son, and I want to thank my wife, Sarah, for encouraging me to continue to work on the book and the show when I just wanted to stay home with her and Cooper. I love you both so much.

Finally, Colin, Woody, James, Cabell, and Page at Clutter Cleaner are all truly my brothers. From our very first house to whatever adventures lie ahead of us, I am proud of the men they have become. A special thanks to our clients, who have taught me so much by sharing their deepest thoughts and secrets with the crew and me. Their stories and lessons will live on in this book and help other families understand, heal, and grow.

INDEX

Page numbers in *italics* indicate photographs; those in **bold** indicate charts.

THE SECRET LIVES OF HOARDERS

THE SECRET LIVES OF HOARDERS

THE SECRET LIVES OF HOARDERS

THE SECRET LIVES OF HOARDERS

THE SECRET LIVES OF HOARDERS

THE SECRET LIVES OF HOARDERS

THE SECRET LIVES OF HOARDERS

ABOUT THE AUTHORS

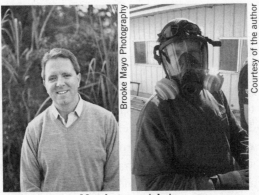

Brooke Mayo Photography

Courtesy of the author

Matt, between jobs!

With his company, Clutter Cleaner, **Matt Paxton** is a featured hoarder specialist on A&E's *Hoarders*. He appears regularly on radio and television, where he speaks on hoarding and senior relocation.

Paxton has been, variously, a research analyst, a database manager for Caesar's Palace, a triathlon wetsuit designer, a professional gambler, a volunteer grief counselor for children, and a housecleaner. He has started three companies, traveled around the world, and run five marathons. When Paxton started Clutter Cleaner in 2006, it was intended to focus on organizing and cleaning houses for grieving widows and relocating seniors, but he quickly found himself sought out by extreme hoarders.

Paxton went to college at the University of Mary Washington, where he earned a degree in business administration.

As a teenager he spent time with his great-aunt, who had a serious hoarding problem. He estimates he cleaned her house at least twenty times while he was growing up. Today, he and his wife, Sarah, live in that house in Richmond, Virginia, with their son and dog. It is very clean.

To learn more about hoarding and to follow Matt, visit his website at www.5decisionsaway.com.

Phaedra Hise has covered subjects including entrepreneurship, small aircraft accidents, big problems raising kids, and what it feels like to rev a motorcycle around a racetrack at over 100 mph. She is an instrument-rated private pilot, a triathlete, a competitive cyclist, a scuba diver, and the cofounder of a growing literary nonprofit, and was an insider on two company startups.

Her award-winning work has been anthologized and published in national magazines including *AARP*, *Salon*, *Popular Mechanics*, and *Ladies' Home Journal*, and she has covered the world of entrepreneurship as a staff writer for *Inc.* and contributor to the *Wall Street Journal* and *Fortune Small Business*. She has written four other books and lives with her very messy teenaged daughter in Richmond, Virginia.